# REVIEW OF
# Medical Embryology

# 6th

# REVIEW OF
# *Medical*
# *Embryology*

**Keith L. Moore**, **PhD, FIAC, FRSM**

Professor Emeritus, Division of Anatomy, Department of Surgery,
Faculty of Medicine, University of Toronto, Toronto, Ontario, Canada

Former Professor and Head, Department of Anatomy,
University of Manitoba

and former Professor and Chairman,
Department of Anatomy and Cell Biology, University of Toronto

**T.V.N. Persaud**, **MD, PhD, DSc, FRCPath (Lond.)**

Professor Emeritus and Former Head,
Department of Human Anatomy and Cell Science,
Professor of Pediatrics and Child Health, Professor of Obstetrics, Gynecology,
and Reproductive Sciences, Faculty of Medicine, University of Manitoba,

Consultant in Pathology and Clinical Genetics, Health Sciences Centre,
Winnipeg, Manitoba, Canada

Visiting Professor, St. George's University Medical School,
Grenada, West Indies

**SAUNDERS**
An Imprint of Elsevier Science

SAUNDERS
An Imprint of Elsevier Science

The Curtis Center
Independence Square West
Philadelphia, Pennsylvania 19106-3399

REVIEW OF MEDICAL EMBRYOLOGY                    ISBN: 0-2216-0131-6

---

**Notice**

Medical Assisting is an ever-changing field. Standard safety precautions must be followed but as new research and clinical experience broaden our knowledge, changes in treatment and drug therapy may become necessary or appropriate. Readers are advised to check the most current product information provided by the manufacturer of each drug to be administered to verify recommended dose, the method and duration of administration, and contraindications. It is the responsibility of the treating physician, relying on experience and knowledge of the patient, to determine dosages and the best treatment for each individual patient. Neither the Publisher nor the author assume any liability for any injury and/or damage to persons or property arising from this publication.

The Publisher

---

**Library of Congress Cataloging-in-Publication Data**

Moore, Keith L.
    Review of medical embryology/Keith L. Moore, T.V.N. Persaud.–6th ed.
      p.cm.
    ISBN 0-7216-0131-6
        1. Embryology, Human–Examinations, questions, etc. 2. Embryology, Human–Outlines, syllabi, etc. 1. Persaud, T.V.N. II. Title.
QM601.M764 2003
612.6'4–dc21                                                    2002021798

*Acquisition Editor:* Jason Malley

RDC/MVB

Printed in the United States

Last digit is the print number:  9   8   7   6   5   4   3   2   1

*To our wives, children,
and grandchildren*

# User's Guide

This *Review of Medical Embryology* is designed to help you learn and later review human embryology and teratology by providing learning objectives and various types of multiple-choice questions based on these objectives. The guide is not intended as a substitute for careful study of your textbook and lecture notes; however, it is designed to enable you to detect areas of weakness and afford you the opportunity to correct deficits in your knowledge.

Although the answers to the questions are explained and relevant notes are given, you should consult your textbook for a comprehensive review of difficult concepts and processes. Through discussion of weak areas with your colleagues and instructors, you can test your ability to do the things listed as learning objectives. To use this review most effectively, the following steps are suggested:

1. Read the objectives listed at the beginning of the chapter you plan to review.

2. Carefully study the appropriate chapter in your textbook, focusing on the topics included in the objectives.

3. Attempt to answer the questions. All questions are designed to be answered at the rate of about one per minute. As you complete each set of questions, check your answers. If any of your answers are wrong, read the notes and explanations and study the appropriate material and illustrations in your textbook before proceeding to the next set of questions.

4. If you get 80% or more of the questions correct on the first trial, or during a subsequent review, you have performed well and should have no difficulty answering similar questions based on the objectives given in this guide.

# Preface

The sixth edition of this *Review of Medical Embryology* has been thoroughly revised. It is designed primarily for use with the authors' textbooks: *The Developing Human: Clinically Oriented Embryology* and *Before We Are Born: Essentials of Embryology and Birth Defects*, published by the W.B. Saunders Company; however; this review can be used with similar advantage by students using other textbooks of human embryology. The questions deal with the essentials of human embryology and birth defects that are of practical value and are similar to those commonly used in national board examinations such as the USMLE Step 1.

This book is designed as a *study guide for beginning students* and as a *review manual for advanced students* preparing for National Board of Medical Examiners USMLE and other examinations. Because multiple-choice examinations are used more and more, and are formidable even to the best prepared, commonly used types of these questions have been developed around each topic in embryology and teratology. The test questions are intended for those who wish to determine the state of their knowledge and to improve their skills with multiple-choice examinations. More clinically oriented questions and illustrations have been added to this edition.

With less time available for formal study of embryology, there is a need for more independent study by students. To learn independently, stated objectives are required. At the beginning of each chapter, there is a list of objectives indicating what students should be able to do when they have completed their study of the chapter. The self-assessment questions and answers in each chapter provide students with feedback as to their status in achieving the objectives and afford them the opportunity to correct deficits that may exist in their knowledge.

The letters and comments we have received from students around the world expressing their appreciation of this review encouraged us to update the book and add new questions. We are grateful to our students and colleagues for their help in improving the questions and answers. We welcome suggestions for new questions and improvement of old ones. We would like to thank Dr. Mark Torchia, Department of Surgery and Department of Human Anatomy and Cell Science, University of Manitoba; and Professor T. S. Ranganathan, Department of Anatomical Sciences, St. George's University School of Medicine, Grenada, West Indies, for their invaluable contributions. We are especially grateful to Mrs. Marion Moore who has provided editorial assistance with this and previous editions.

KEITH L. MOORE
VID PERSAUD

# Contents

# Introduction to Human Embryology and Teratology

1

## Objectives

Be able to:

- Define the term development and discuss the developmental periods.
- Differentiate between the terms conceptus and abortus.
- Explain why embryology forms a basis for medical and dental practice, including the allied health sciences.
- Differentiate between the terms embryology and teratology.
- Discuss the various terms of position and direction, and illustrate the various planes of the body.
- Explain the difference in meaning between embryo and fetus, conception and conceptus, and embryology and developmental anatomy.

## *Five-Choice Completion Questions*

**Directions:** Each of the following statements or questions is followed by five suggested responses or completions. **Select the one best answer** in each case.

1. The term conceptus includes all structures that develop from the
   - A. chorion
   - B. embryoblast
   - C. zygote
   - D. trophoblast
   - E. inner cell mass

2. Select the best term for describing the foot with reference to the leg.
   - A. distal
   - B. ventral
   - C. posterior
   - D. inferior
   - E. proximal

3. A section through an embryo that divides it into ventral and dorsal parts is a _____ section.
   - A. cross
   - B. sagittal
   - C. frontal
   - D. oblique
   - E. median

4. In the adult, the neck is superior to the thorax. The corresponding term in the fetus is
   - A. dorsal
   - B. inferior
   - C. caudal
   - D. ventral
   - E. cranial

5. The plane that divides a fetus into right and left halves is called the _____ plane.
    A. sagittal
    B. median
    C. coronal
    D. transverse
    E. frontal

6. Which of the following embryological terms means toward the nose?
    A. dorsal
    B. cephalic
    C. cranial
    D. rostral
    E. caudal

7. Which of the following terms of comparison is used incorrectly?
    A. The wrist is distal to the forearm.
    B. The brain is cranial to the spinal cord.
    C. The upper limb arises caudal to the heart.
    D. The knee is proximal to the ankle.
    E. The tail-like eminence of the embryo is caudal to the abdomen.

8. From which of the following is the morula formed?
    A. oocyte
    B. sperm
    C. zygote
    D. blastocyst
    E. gastrula

9. Which of the following statements concerning an abortion is incorrect?
    A. Pregnancy loss may occur during the embryonic period.
    B. Pregnancy loss may occur after the eighth week of gestation.
    C. The aborted embryo is not viable.
    D. The conceptus is always expelled from the uterus.
    E. Abortion may be clinically induced.

## Answers and Explanations

1. **C**   The term conceptus is used when referring to the embryo (or fetus) and its membranes (i.e., the total products of conception that develop from the zygote). The conceptus (embryo and its membranes) that is expelled or removed during an abortion is called an abortus.

2. **A**   The foot is at the distal end of the leg. The term distal is commonly used in descriptions of a limb instead of the term inferior.

3. **C**   A vertical section through the frontal plane is known as a frontal (coronal) section.

4. **E**   The neck of a fetus is cranial to the thorax; that is, it is closer to the head. Cranial means toward the cranium.

5. **B**   The median plane is the vertical plane that passes through the center of the body, dividing it into right and left halves. There is only one median plane.

6. **D**   The term rostral is used to indicate the relation of structures to the nose (L. *rostrum*, a beak). For example, the philtrum of the lip is rostral to the eye.

7. **C**   The upper limb arises opposite the heart. The Latin term *caudal* means toward the caudal eminence.

8. **C**   Cleavage, or division, of the zygote gives rise to a ball of blastomeres, called a morula. Cleavage occurs about 3 days after fertilization

and precedes the formation of the blastocyst and the gastrula.

9. **D** Termination of pregnancy, whether naturally occurring or clinically induced, before 20 weeks of gestation is an abortion. The aborted embryo is not viable. In cases of missed abortion the products of conception are not expelled from the uterus. Spontaneous abortions occur naturally during the first 12 weeks of pregnancy; many are not detected clinically, especially when they occur very early in pregnancy.

# Five-Choice Association Questions

**Directions:** Each group of questions below consists of a numbered list of descriptive words or phrases accompanied by a diagram with certain parts indicated by letters or by a list of lettered headings. For each numbered word or phrase, **select the lettered part of the heading** that matches it correctly and then insert the letter in the space to the right of the appropriate number. Sometimes more than one numbered word or phrase may be correctly matched to the same lettered part or heading.

A. Median
B. Dorsal
C. Frontal

D. Caudal
E. Rostral

1. _____ Posterior
2. _____ Toward nose
3. _____ Coronal

4. _____ Midsagittal
5. _____ Toward "tail"
6. _____ Lying in middle

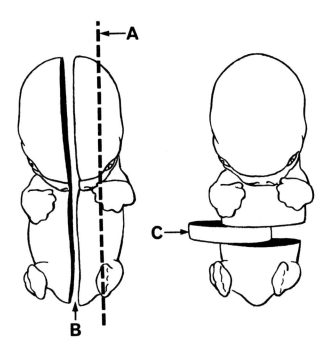
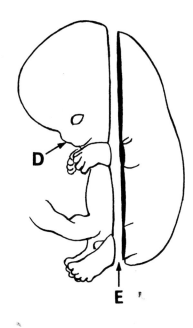

7. _____ Transverse plane
8. _____ Rostral
9. _____ Median plane

10. _____ Frontal plane
11. _____ Sagittal plane

## Answers and Explanations

1. **B**  Dorsal refers to structures near the posterior surface or back. In the adult, dorsal is equivalent to posterior. The term dorsal is used in descriptions of embryos and in some descriptions of embryos and in some terms of adults (e.g., we refer to the dorsum or the dorsal part of the foot and hand).

2. **E**  Structures that are near the nose or oral region are rostral (e.g., a structure such as a nerve grows rostrally (toward the nose or nasal region) or in a rostral direction).

3. **C**  The term coronal often is used synonymously with frontal. Coronal refers to the fact that a coronal plane passes through the coronal suture of the cranium.

4. **A**  A midsagittal section passes through the median plane. Thus, the terms midsagittal and median are used synonymously in reference to sections cut in the median plane, but the term median is preferable.

5. **D**  Caudal is used in the description of structures that are near the caudal eminence ("tail") of the embryo. Embryos have tail-like structures until the early part of the eighth week. In descriptions of adult anatomy, the term inferior is used to indicate structures that are lower in the body (e.g., the large intestine is inferior to the stomach).

6. **A**  Median means lying in the median plane or midline, and the term medial is used to indicate a structure nearer the median plane (e.g., the eye is medial to the auricle of the external ear).

7. **C**  The transverse plane is any plane that is at right angles to both the median and frontal planes. The term transverse often is used synonymously with horizontal. Transverse implies that it is through the longitudinal axis of a structure. In the anatomical position, a transverse section through the foot in the anatomical position is in the frontal plane.

8. **D**  The term rostral (toward the nose or nasal region) is used to indicate the relation of a structure to the nose (e.g., the eyes are rostral to the ears).

9. **B**  The median plane is a vertical plane that passes through the center of the body, dividing it into right and left halves. Median sections of embryos show the relation of thoracic and abdominal structures to each other.

10. **E**  A frontal plane is any vertical plane that intersects the median plane at a right angle. This kind of section is helpful in studying paired structures (e.g., the kidneys).

11. **A**  A sagittal plane is any vertical plane that passes through the body parallel to the median plane. A median section passes through the median plane. These sections often are used to show the course of structures that run through various regions of the body (e.g., the esophagus runs through the neck and thorax).

# The Beginning of Human Development

**2**

## Objectives

Be able to:

- Describe spermatogenesis and oogenesis with emphasis on the chromosomal changes that occur.
- Compare the sperm and oocyte with reference to size, chromosome constitution, time of formation, transport, and viability.
- Define the term nondisjunction, and explain how this abnormal process leads to monosomy and trisomy. Describe the most common syndrome that results from nondisjunction.
- Discuss the ovarian cycle and the menstrual cycle, explaining how ovarian cyclic activity is intimately linked with cyclic changes in the endometrium.
- Discuss capacitation and the acrosome reaction of the sperm.
- List the results of fertilization.
- Discuss cleavage of the zygote and implantation of the blastocyst, using labeled sketches. Define blastocyst, zona pellucida, trophoblast, inner cell mass, blastocystic cavity, embryonic pole, embryoblast, and hypoblast.

## Five-Choice Completion Questions

**Directions:** Each of the following statements or questions is followed by five suggested responses or completions. **Select the one best answer** in each case.

1. Before ejaculation, sperm are stored chiefly in the
   - A. seminal glands
   - B. efferent ductules
   - C. ejaculatory ducts
   - D. epididymis
   - E. rete testis

2. Which of the following types of germ cell does not undergo cell division?
   - A. spermatogonia
   - B. primary oocytes
   - C. spermatids
   - D. secondary spermatocytes
   - E. oogonia

3. Which of the following chromosomal constitutions in a sperm normally results in a male embryo, if it fertilizes an oocyte (ovum)?
   - A. 22, O
   - B. 22, X
   - C. 22, Y
   - D. 23, X
   - E. 23, Y

4. Oogonia divide by mitosis during
   A. all postnatal periods
   B. early fetal life
   C. puberty
   D. the reproductive period
   E. embryogenesis

5. The normal chromosome number of a human spermatid is
   A. 23 autosomes plus 2 different sex chromosomes
   B. 22 autosomes plus an X and a Y chromosome
   C. 23 autosomes plus 2 identical sex chromosomes
   D. 22 autosomes plus an X or a Y chromosome
   E. 46, XY

6. Morphologically abnormal sperm may cause
   A. monosomy
   B. congenital anomalies
   C. trisomy
   D. abnormal embryos
   E. infertility

7. Which of the following layers of the embryo is recognizable at the end of the first week of development?
   A. hypoblast
   B. mesoderm
   C. ectoderm
   D. splanchnopleure
   E. somatopleure

8. The secondary oocyte completes the second meiotic division
   A. before ovulation
   B. during ovulation
   C. at fertilization
   D. before birth
   E. at puberty

9. Sperms penetrate the zona pellucida, digesting a path by the action of enzymes released from its _____ .
   A. middle piece
   B. acrosome
   C. neck
   D. main piece
   E. head

10. How many sperms would probably be deposited by a normal young adult male in the vagina during sexual intercourse?
    A. 300 thousand
    B. 3 million
    C. 30 million
    D. 300 million
    E. 3 billion

11. A 42-year-old woman became pregnant. She was concerned about the health of her unborn child and consulted a physician. There is a risk for which of the following?
    A. intrauterine growth retardation
    B. gene mutation
    C. chromosomal abnormalities
    D. miscarriage
    E. premature birth

12. Freshly ejaculated sperms are not capable of fertilizing oocytes because these sperms are:
    A. inactive
    B. not capacitated
    C. morphologically abnormal
    D. immature
    E. very motile

13. An ultrasound examination of a pregnant woman revealed the presence of 7 embryos. Which of the following is the probable cause?
    A. The embroblast divided into 7 embryos.
    B. Progesterone secretion is increased.
    C. The woman was treated with an antifertility drug.
    D. Seven oocytes were fertilized by 7 sperms.
    E. Release of gonadotropins is inadequate.

14. The semen of a man believed to be responsible for a sterile marriage was evaluated. Which of the following is of least importance in assessing the man's fertility?
    A. sperm count
    B. sperm morphology
    C. zinc concentration
    D. calcium ions
    E. sperm motility

15. During spermatogenesis, which of the following cells undergo a second meiotic division?
    A. spermatogonia
    B. primary spermatocytes
    C. secondary spermatocytes
    D. spermatids
    E. sperms

16. An infant is diagnosed as having 47 chromosomes instead of 46. This abnormal condition (trisomy) results from
    A. gene mutation
    B. nondisjunction
    C. disturbances in spermiogenesis
    D. disturbances in mitosis
    E. abnormal spermatogonia

## Answers and Explanations

1. **D**  Sperms are stored and undergo further maturation in the epididymis. They are not normally stored in the seminal glands (vesicles), as was believed for many years. During ejaculation, the sperms are forced through the ductus deferens into the urethra, from which they are expelled with the secretions of the accessory glands (e.g., the prostate) as semen. If not ejaculated, the sperms degenerate and are absorbed within the epididymis.

2. **C**  Spermatids do not divide. They are gradually transformed into mature sperms during spermiogenesis.

3. **E**  Fertilization of a secondary oocyte (ovum) by a Y sperm (i.e., 23, Y) produces a 46, XY zygote that normally develops into a male. The number 46 designates the total number of chromosomes, including the two sex chromosomes (XY). The sex of an embryo depends on whether an X or a Y sperm fertilizes the oocyte. The mother can contribute only an X chromosome and so cannot determine the embryo's sex.

4. **B**  Oogonia proliferate during the early fetal period and, unlike spermatogonia, do not increase at puberty. All oogonia become primary oocytes before birth. Many of the 2 million or so oocytes present in both ovaries at birth degenerate before puberty, leaving about 40,000 to undergo further development after puberty.

5. **D**  Spermatids are haploid cells (23 chromosomes) that have 22 autosomes plus a Y or an X chromosome (i.e., one or the other but not both). Thus, the haploid number in humans is 23. If two members of a chromosome pair fail to separate (nondisjunction), abnormal spermatids can have 22 autosomes and 2 sex chromosomes, or no sex chromosome.

6. **E**  Structurally abnormal sperms do not fertilize oocytes because of their lack of normal motility and fertilizing power. Examination of semen is important in the study of fertility. The number, motility, and abnormalities in size and shape of sperms are important in assessing sterility in males. If 20% or more sperms are morphologically abnormal, fertility usually is impaired.

7. **A**  The bilaminar embryonic disc forms early in the second week. At the end of the first week, the hypoblast (primordial endoderm) begins to form on the ventral surface of the embryoblast (inner cell mass) from the inner cell mass by delamination.

8. **C**  When a sperm contacts the cell membrane of a secondary oocyte, the oocyte completes the second maturation or meiotic division and becomes a mature oocyte (ovum). The second polar body, a nonfunctional cell, is formed during this division. If fertilization does not occur, the secondary oocyte does not complete this division; it degenerates within 24 hours after ovulation.

9. **B**  A sperm digests a path for itself through the corona radiata and zona pellucida by the action of enzymes released from the sperm's acrosome through perforations that develop in it during the acrosome reaction. Acrosomal enzymes, especially acrosin, are also important for the penetration of the zona pellucida.

10. **D**  At least 300 million sperms are deposited in the vagina during sexual intercourse. Usually 200 million to 600 million sperms are in the ejaculate, but only a few hundred sperms are believed to reach the fertilization site. If less than 50 million sperms are present in a semen sample, the male from whom the sample was taken may be infertile.

11. **C**  The incidence of children with trisomy 21 or Down syndrome increases with maternal age. Because of the woman's age, the primary oocytes have been dormant in arrested first meiotic division for about 30 years. During meiosis, sometimes homologous chromosomes fail to separate and migrate to opposite poles of the cell, a condition known as nondisjunction.

The result is that some germ cells have 24 chromosomes instead of 23, and others have only 22. Trisomy occurs when a gamete with 24 chromosomes fuses with a normal one during fertilization, forming a zygote with 47 chromosomes.

12. **B**  Glycoproteins and seminal proteins on the surface of the acrosome of freshly ejaculated sperms must first be removed to facilitate fertilization of the oocyte. This process, which lasts about 7 hours, is known as capacitation and usually occurs in the uterus. Capacitated sperms are more active.

13. **D**  The woman probably was treated with fertility drugs (e.g., gonadotropins) to stimulate ovulation. The incidence of multiple pregnancy increases considerably when ovulation is stimulated. The large number of embryos present probably resulted from the fertilization of many mature oocytes by individual sperms.

14. **C**  Zinc concentrations of the male reproductive organs are relatively high, but there is no difference in zinc concentrations of semen (seminal fluid) from fertile and infertile men. In normal males, there are more than 100 million sperms per milliliter of semen. Less than 10 million sperms per milliliter of semen are likely to be from someone who is sterile, especially if there are immotile and abnormal sperms in the specimen. Calcium ions in the semen, like prostaglandins, are involved in the movement of sperms.

15. **C**  Secondary spermatocytes undergo a second meiotic division to form spermatids, which subsequently are transformed into mature sperms. Spermatogonia grow and give rise to the primary spermatocytes by mitotic division. Each primary spermatocyte then undergoes the first meiotic division to form two secondary spermatocytes with a haploid chromosomal complement.

16. **B**  Trisomy is a relatively common numerical chromosomal anomaly resulting from an error in meiotic cell division during gametogenesis. When homologous chromosomes fail to separate and migrate to opposite poles of the germ cell, some gametes have 24 chromosomes and

others have 22. This abnormal condition is known as *nondisjunction*. In the event of fertilization occurring between a gamete with 24 chromosomes and a normal gamete with 23 chromosomes, the resulting zygote has 47 chromosomes (trisomy). Spermatogonia are the primordial male germ cells with a chromosomal constitution of 46, XY. Spermatids differentiate into mature sperms during spermiogenesis.

## Five-Choice Association Questions

**Directions:** Each group of questions below consists of a numbered list of descriptive words or phrases accompanied by a diagram with certain parts indicated by letters or by a list of lettered headings. For each numbered word or phrase, **select the lettered part or heading** that matches it correctly and then insert the letter in the space to the right of the appropriate number. Sometimes more than one numbered word or phrase may be correctly matched to the same lettered part or heading.

A. Polar body
B. Capacitation
C. Acrosome

D. Zona pellucida
E. Pronuclei

1. _____ Haploid nuclei that fuse to form a zygote
2. _____ Changes occur in it that inhibit entry of sperm
3. _____ Contains enzymes that digest a path for the sperm
4. _____ Nonfunctional cell produced during oogenesis

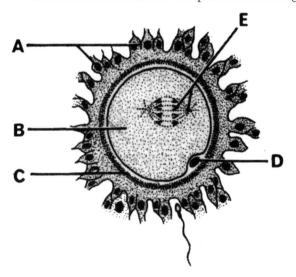

5. _____ Polar body
6. _____ Zona pellucida
7. _____ Diploid cells
8. _____ Meiotic spindle
9. _____ Corona radiata
10. _____ Haploid cell

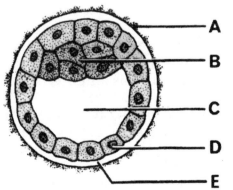

11. _____ Embryoblast
12. _____ Gives rise to part of placenta
13. _____ Gives rise to the embryo
14. _____ Gives rise to the hypoblast
15. _____ Degenerates and disappears
16. _____ Blastocystic cavity

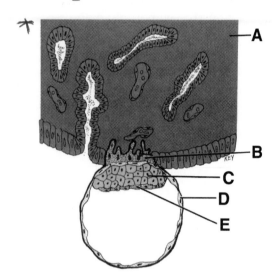

17. _____ Once filled cavity of ovarian follicle
18. _____ Develops under luteinizing hormone influence
19. _____ Produces progesterone
20. _____ Expelled with the follicular fluid
21. _____ Fimbriae
22. _____ Derived from a primary oocyte

23. _____ Cytotrophoblast
24. _____ Embryoblast
25. _____ Endometrium
26. _____ Hypoblast
27. _____ Syncytiotrophoblast

## Answers and Explanations

1. **E**  The male and female pronuclei are the haploid nuclei of the sperm and oocyte, respectively. They fuse during fertilization to form the diploid nucleus of a zygote. The nucleus occupies most of the head of the sperm, and after it enters the oocyte, it swells to form the male pronucleus. The pronuclei are about equal in size and show similar features.

2. **D**  The zona pellucida undergoes changes, called the zona reaction, when a sperm contacts the cell membrane of a secondary oocyte. These changes, caused by the release of substances from the oocyte, prevent other sperms from passing through the zona pellucida and entering the oocyte.

3. **C**  The acrosome is a caplike structure that invests the anterior half of the head of the sperm. It contains enzymes that pass through perforations in its wall and digest a path for the sperm to follow through the zona pellucida to fertilize the oocyte.

4. **A**  The polar body is a small haploid cell produced during the first and second meiotic divisions. Polar bodies have the same number of chromosomes as the secondary and mature oocytes; however, they receive very little cytoplasm. Most cytoplasm goes to the mature oocyte.

5. **D**  The first polar body forms during the first meiotic division. Note that it is inside the zona

pellucida with the secondary oocyte. Although it may divide into two polar bodies, these cells degenerate. The secondary oocyte receives the same number of chromosomes as the polar body; however, it gets almost all the cytoplasm.

6. **C** The zona pellucida surrounds the secondary oocyte and the polar body. This membrane is surrounded by a layer of follicular cells called the corona radiata. The zona pellucida appears homogeneous in the fresh condition, but under the electron microscope it appears granular and shows some concentric layering.

7. **A** The follicular cells of the corona radiata are the only diploid cells in the diagram. During follicular development, the follicular cells proliferate by mitosis and form a stratified epithelium around the oocyte. In the mature follicle, the oocyte lies in a mound of follicular cells, called the cumulus oophorus. When the oocyte is expelled at ovulation, it is surrounded by the zona pellucida and one or more layers of follicular cells, as shown in the diagram.

8. **E** Contact of a sperm with the cell membrane of the oocyte stimulates the secondary oocyte to complete its second meiotic division. This contact also brings about the zona reaction, preventing entry of more sperms. The sperm penetrates the cell membrane of the secondary oocyte and then passes into the cytoplasm of the oocyte, leaving its cell membrane outside the oocyte.

9. **A** The corona radiata consists of one or more layers of follicular cells that surround the zona pellucida, the polar body, and the secondary oocyte. The corona radiata is dispersed during fertilization by enzymes released from the acrosomes of the sperms that surround the oocyte.

10. **D** The polar body is the labelled haploid cell formed during the first meiotic division of the oocyte. The sperm is also a haploid cell zygote.

11. **B** The embryoblast (inner cell mass) is recognizable about 4 days after fertilization. It is derived from the central cells of the morula. The embryoblast gives rise to the embryo and some extraembryonic tissues.

12. **D** The trophoblast gives rise to the embryonic part of the placenta; the other part is derived from the endometrium. When the trophoblast becomes lined by extraembryonic somatic mesoderm, the combined layers are called the chorion. The trophoblast forms no part of the embryo.

13. **B** The embryoblast gives rise to the embryo. The first sign of differentiation of the cells of the embryoblast is the appearance of the hypoblast on its ventral surface. The embryoblast later gives rise to two more germ layers. The three germ layers give rise to all the tissues and organs of the embryo.

14. **B** At the end of the first week, differentiation of the embryoblast gives rise to the hypoblast. It appears as a flattened layer on the ventral surface of the inner cell mass. Later, it forms the roof of the yolk sac and is incorporated into the embryo as the lining of the primordial gut.

15. **A** The zona pellucida begins to degenerate about 4 days after fertilization as the blastocyst begins to expand rapidly. Implantation of the blastocyst begins on the sixth day.

16. **C** The blastocystic cavity forms as fluid passes into the morula from the uterus and accumulates. The spaces around the central cells of the morula coalesce to form the blastocystic cavity, converting the morula into a blastocyst. The uterine fluid in the blastocystic cavity bathes the ventral surface of the embryoblast and probably supplies nutrients to the embryonic cells.

17. **C** Follicular fluid fills the cavities of mature ovarian follicles. When the stigma of the follicle ruptures at ovulation, the oocyte is expelled with the fluid from the follicle and the ovary in a few seconds. The expulsion of the oocyte and the fluid is the result of intrafollicular pressure and, possibly, ovarian smooth muscle contraction.

18. **E** The corpus luteum develops under the influence of the luteinizing hormone. It produces progesterone and some estrogen. These hormones act on the endometrium, bringing

about the secretory phase and preparing the endometrium for implantation of a blastocyst. If the oocyte is fertilized, the corpus luteum enlarges into a corpus luteum of pregnancy and increases its hormone production. If the ovum is not fertilized, the corpus luteum begins to degenerate about 9 days after ovulation and is called a corpus luteum of menstruation.

19. **E**   The corpus luteum usually produces progesterone for about 9 days. If the oocyte is fertilized, it produces progesterone until about the end of the fourth month of pregnancy.

20. **B**   The secondary oocyte is expelled with follicular fluid at ovulation. Ovulation is under FSH and LH influence and occurs through the ruptured stigma. The oocyte quickly leaves the peritoneal cavity and enters the infundibulum of the uterine tube.

21. **D**   The fimbriae of the uterine tube embrace the ovary at ovulation. The sweeping motion of the fimbriae and the motion of the cilia on their epithelial lining cells carry the oocyte into the uterine tube.

22. **B**   The secondary oocyte is derived from a primary oocyte after the first meiotic division. This division produces two haploid cells, the secondary oocyte and the first polar body. By the time of ovulation, the secondary oocyte has begun the second meiotic division but progresses only to the metaphase stage, where division is arrested. If the oocyte is fertilized, it completes the division, forming a mature oocyte.

23. **D**   The trophoblast of the implanting blastocyst differentiates into two layers. The internal layer is the cytotrophoblast. Rapid proliferation of cells of the cytotrophoblast give rise to the syncytiotrophoblast, a nucleated cytoplasmic mass.

24. **C**   The embryoblast gives rise to the embryo. It arises from cells that have segregated from the morula. This occurs about 4 days after fertilization. The remaining cells of the morula become the trophoblast of the blastocyst.

25. **A**   The blastocyst attaches to the epithelium covering the compact layer of the endometrium about 6 days after fertilization. The endometrium is in the secretory phase of the uterine cycle, with abundant blood vessels and secreting glands. The endometrial cells are enlarged and filled with glycogen as well as lipids.

26. **E**   The hypoblast appears at about 7 days after fertilization. It is a flattened layer of cells on the surface of the inner cell mass facing the blastocyst cavity. The hypoblast gives rise to the embryonic endoderm and the endoderm of the yolk sac.

27. **B**   The syncytiotrophoblast, like the cytotrophoblast, is derived from the trophoblast. The trophoblast proliferates rapidly following implantation of the blastocyst. The syncytiotrophoblast is a multinucleated cytoplasmic mass with no discernible cell boundaries. The syncytiotrophoblast invades the uterine endometrium and facilitates implantation of the blastocyst.

# Formation of Bilaminar Embryonic Disc and Chorionic Sac

**3**

## Objectives

Be able to:

- Describe implantation of a blastocyst using simple labeled diagrams.
- Discuss proliferation and differentiation of the trophoblast, formation of lacunar networks, and the establishment of the primordial uteroplacental circulation.
- Trace the development of the amniotic cavity, bilaminar embryonic disc, yolk sac, extraembryonic mesoderm, extraembryonic coelom, and connecting stalk.
- Define these terms: the prechordal plate, embryotroph, chorion, primary chorionic villi, chorionic sac, decidual reaction, and ectopic pregnancies.

## Five-Choice Completion Questions

**Directions:** Each of the following statements or questions is followed by five suggested responses or completions. **Select the one best answer** in each case.

1. The 8-day blastocyst
   - A. has a single layer of trophoblast at the embryonic pole
   - B. has lacunae in the syncytiotrophoblast
   - C. is partially implanted in the endometrium
   - D. is covered by the uterine epithelium
   - E. has a primary yolk sac

2. The syncytiotrophoblast
   - A. surrounds the 8-day blastocyst
   - B. has well-defined cell boundaries
   - C. shows little invasive activity
   - D. is derived from cytotrophoblast
   - E. is nonfunctional

3. The amniotic cavity develops
   - A. initially on the 10th day
   - B. within the exocoelomic cavity
   - C. between the embryonic disc and trophoblast
   - D. in the extraembryonic mesoderm
   - E. during the first week

**13**

4. A blastocyst of about two-weeks' gestation was found in a gynecological specimen sent to the laboratory for examination. Which of the following is a characteristic feature of a blastocyst at about this age?
   A. presence of primary chorionic villi
   B. incompletely implanted in the endometrium
   C. notochord is present
   D. intraembryonic coelom surrounds the yolk sac
   E. gastrulation is in progress

5. In the 10- to 12-day blastocyst
   A. the conceptus lies deep to the endometrial epithelium
   B. the defect in the endometrial epithelium is indicated by a closing plug
   C. the implanted blastocyst produces an elevation on the endometrial surface
   D. maternal blood begins to flow slowly through the lacunar networks
   E. all the above are correct

6. The wall of the chorionic sac is composed of
   A. cytotrophoblast and syncytiotrophoblast
   B. two layers of trophoblast lined by extraembryonic somatic mesoderm
   C. trophoblast and the exocoelomic membrane
   D. extraembryonic splanchnic mesoderm and both layers of trophoblast
   E. none of the above is correct

7. During the second week, lacunar networks develop within the
   A. extraembryonic mesoderm          D. endometrium
   B. outer cell mass                  E. embryoblast
   C. syncytiotrophoblast

8. Ectopic implantations most commonly occur in the
   A. ovary                            D. peritoneal cavity
   B. abdomen                          E. cervix
   C. uterine tube

9. Implantation of the blastocyst
   A. inhibits the decidual reaction
   B. is controlled by progesterone
   C. occurs in the stratum spongiosum
   D. involves invasion of the endometrium by cytotrophoblast
   E. usually occurs on the anterior wall of the uterus

10. The amniotic cavity appears on the eighth day as a slitlike space between the trophoblast and the
    A. extraembryonic mesoderm          D. connecting stalk
    B. embryoblast                      E. chorion
    C. exocoelomic membrane

11. A 32-year-old woman was admitted to hospital because of low abdominal pain and hemorrhage. Her last menstrual period was about 7 weeks earlier. Which of the following is the most likely diagnosis?
    A. appendicitis                     D. ectopic pregnancy
    B. ovarian cyst                     E. placenta previa
    C. miscarriage

12. Which of the following structures is formed during the second week of development?
    A. notochord
    B. neural plate
    C. intraembryonic coelom
    D. somite
    E. chorionic sac

## Answers and Explanations

1. **C**  The 8-day blastocyst is partially implanted in the endometrium. The trophoblast at the abembryonic pole opposite the embryonic pole remains relatively undifferentiated, consisting of a thin layer of cytotrophoblastic cells. The trophoblast consists of two layers only where it is in contact with the endometrium (usually adjacent to the embryoblast). The primary yolk sac is not usually present at 8 days, but the amniotic cavity is represented by a slitlike space.

2. **D**  The syncytiotrophoblast is derived from the cytotrophoblast. This cellular layer is mitotically active and forms new cells that fuse with and become part of the increasing mass of syncytiotrophoblast. The syncytiotrophoblast does not enclose the 8-day blastocyst on all sides. It forms a multinucleated cytoplasmic mass at the embryonic pole. The syncytiotrophoblast does not have well-defined cell boundaries. Invasiveness is one of the spectacular properties of the syncytiotrophoblast. The penetration and subsequent erosion of the endometrium by the syncytiotrophoblast results from proteolytic enzymes produced by the syncytiotrophoblast.

3. **C**  The amniotic cavity appears as a small cavity in the embryoblast on the eighth day after fertilization between the embryonic disc and the invading syncytiotrophoblast. It does not develop in the exocoelomic cavity or in the extraembryonic mesoderm. The amnion forms from cells derived from the epiblast.

4. **A**  Primary chorionic villi are characteristic features of the 14-day blastocyst. All the other statements about the blastocyst at the end of the second week are incorrect. The blastocyst is completely implanted by the end of the second week. The notochord, intraembryonic mesoderm, and intraembryonic coelom are formed during the third week.

5. **E**  All these statements about the 10- to 12-day blastocyst are true. The important statement is **D** because the presence of maternal blood establishes an abundant source of nutrition for the conceptus.

6. **B**  The wall of the chorionic sac is composed of the chorion, which is formed by the combination of extraembryonic somatic mesoderm and the two layers of trophoblast (cytotrophoblast and syncytiotrophoblast). The chorionic sac contains the embryo, which is attached to the wall of the sac by the connecting stalk.

7. **C**  Lacunar networks develop in the syncytiotrophoblast by coalescence of lacunae (spaces). Although spaces or cavities form in the extraembryonic mesoderm, they are not called lacunae and they do not form lacunar networks. These extraembryonic coelomic spaces become confluent to form the extraembryonic coelom.

8. **C**  Ectopic, or extrauterine, pregnancies usually occur in the ampulla of the uterine tube. They are related to factors that delay or prevent passage of the morula to the uterus. Tubal rupture may be followed by early expulsion of the conceptus and secondary implantation of the blastocyst in the mesentery of the intestine, for example. Ectopic pregnancies, other than those in the tube, are rare. Cervical implantations are not ectopic (outside uterus), but they are abnormal.

9. **B**  The stratum spongiosum of the endometrium is not directly involved with early implantation. It does become involved with formation of the placenta later in pregnancy.

The decidual reaction is the series of changes that occur in the endometrium as a result of implantation. It is believed that the blastocyst produces hormone-like substances that cause the decidual changes. Progesterone produced by the corpus luteum is the hormone believed to control implantation. Invasion of the endometrium by the syncytiotrophoblast is the most striking event that occurs during implantation. The trophoblast produces proteolytic enzymes that erode the endometrium. The blastocyst usually implants on the posterior wall of the uterine cavity.

10. **B** The amniotic cavity appears as a space between the trophoblast and the embryoblast. Attachment of the blastocyst to the endometrium usually occurs at the embryonic pole where the embryo is developing.

11. **D** The clinical symptoms, as well as the missed menstrual period, suggest an ectopic pregnancy (i.e., the blastocyst is implanted outside the uterine cavity). More than 90% of ectopic implantations occur in the uterine tubes, the majority in the ampulla or infundibulum. Rupture of the uterine tube and hemorrhage are serious complications.

12. **E** The epiblast and hypoblast of the bilaminar embryonic disc are derived from the embryoblast during the second week of development. The amniotic cavity, yolk sac, connecting stalk, and chorion are also formed during this period of development. The neural plate develops during the third week of development from embryonic ectoderm. The notochord, somites, and intraembryonic coelom are formed during the third week.

# Five-Choice Association Questions

**Directions:** Each group of questions below consists of a numbered list of descriptive words or phrases accompanied by a diagram with certain parts indicated by letters or by a list of lettered headings. For each numbered word or phrase, **select the lettered part or heading** that matches it correctly and then insert the letter in the space to the right of the appropriate number. Sometimes more than one numbered word or phrase may be correctly matched to the same lettered part or heading.

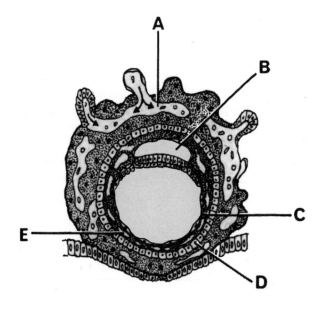

1. _____ Extraembryonic coelom
2. _____ Contains embryotroph
3. _____ Cytotrophoblast
4. _____ Lacunar network
5. _____ Epiblast forms its floor

A. Corpus luteum
B. Zona pellucida
C. Prechordal plate

D. Ectopic implantation
E. Chorionic sac

6. _____ Frequently occurs in uterine tube
7. _____ Develops as a localized thickening of hypoblast
8. _____ Develops from a ruptured ovarian follicle
9. _____ Surrounds embryo, amnion, and yolk sac
10. _____ Enlarges as soon as implantation of a blastocyst occurs

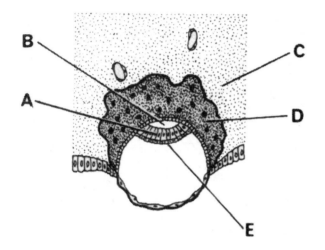

11. _____ Derived from cytotrophoblast
12. _____ Ventral layer of embryonic disc
13. _____ Site of the decidual reaction
14. _____ Multinucleated mass of cytoplasm
15. _____ Lies between the cytotrophoblast and the epiblast

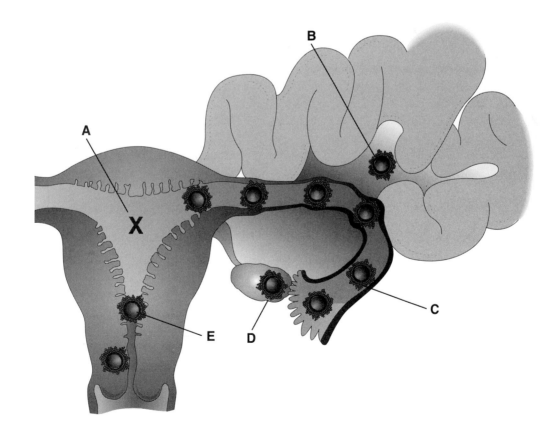

16. _____ Most common site of an ectopic pregnancy
17. _____ Abdominal pregnancy
18. _____ Usual site of implantation
19. _____ Implantation at internal os
20. _____ Ovarian pregnancy

## Answers and Explanations

1. **E**  The extraembryonic coelom, part of which is indicated in the diagram, consists of isolated spaces in the extraembryonic mesoderm. Later, these spaces coalesce to form a single, large cavity.

2. **A**  The lacunar networks (future intervillous spaces) contain a nutrient material known as embryotroph (nutritive material). It is required by the embryo for growth and differentiation. Embryotroph consists of maternal blood, degenerated decidual cells, blood vessels, and glandular tissue.

3. **D**  The cytotrophoblast is the inner layer of the trophoblast. It gives rise to (1) the outer layer of trophoblast (syncytiotrophoblast), (2) amnioblasts (cells that form the amnion), and (3) part of the extraembryonic mesoderm. The cytotrophoblast, as the prefix *cyto* implies, is a cellular layer.

4. **A**  The lacunar networks form by coalescence of lacunae in the syncytiotrophoblast. As the maternal sinusoids are eroded, blood seeps into these networks. Nutrients in the embryotroph diffuse through the two layers of trophoblast and pass to the embryo by way of the extraembryonic coelom.

5. **B**  The floor of the amniotic cavity is formed by the epiblast. The amnion enclosing the amniotic cavity is attached to the epiblast of the embryonic disc. Initially, some amniotic fluid may be secreted by the amniotic cells, but most of it is derived from the maternal blood.

6. **D**  Ectopic implantations usually occur in the uterine tube, most frequently in the ampulla, where fertilization normally occurs. Other sites of ectopic (extrauterine) implantations are in the ovary and on the abdominal peritoneum.

7. **C**  The prechordal plate indicates the future cranial end of the embryo and the future site of the mouth. It is a circular area of endoderm that is firmly adherent to the overlying embryonic epiblast. It is an important landmark in the early embryo and serves as an organizer of the cranial region of the embryo.

8. **A**  The corpus luteum develops from the ovarian follicle after ovulation. Under the influence of luteinizing hormone (LH) produced by the adenohypophysis (anterior lobe of pituitary gland), the ruptured follicle develops into a glandular structure. At ovulation, the walls of the follicle collapse and, with cells of the theca folliculi, form the corpus luteum. The corpus luteum is an important source of progesterone for about 4 months. After this, the placenta is the major producer of this hormone.

9. **E**  The chorion forms the chorionic sac from the wall of which the embryo, its amnion and yolk sac are suspended by the connecting stalk. The chorionic sac gives rise to the embryonic part of the placenta.

10. **A**  If an oocyte is fertilized and the blastocyst implants, the corpus luteum enlarges to form a corpus luteum of pregnancy and increases its production of progesterone. The corpus luteum is an important source of progesterone during the first trimester (90 days); it also produces estrogen. In later pregnancy, these hormones are produced by the placenta.

11. **D**  The syncytiotrophoblast is derived from the cytotrophoblast. Cells of the cytotrophoblast divide mitotically, and some of these cells move outward, where they fuse with and become part of the increasing mass of syncytiotrophoblast. The syncytiotrophoblast produces human chorionic gonadotropin, which acts like luteinizing hormone in maintaining the corpus luteum. Later, it also produces other hormones.

12. **E**  The hypoblast (primordial endoderm) forms the ventral layer of the embryonic disc. It is first recognizable on the ventral surface of the embryoblast about 7 days after fertilization.

13. **C**  The connective tissue in the compact layer of the endometrium in the region of the implanting blastocyst is the site of cellular and

other changes known as the decidual reaction. The enlarged decidual cells contain large amounts of glycogen and lipids that provide nourishment for the embryo.

14. **D** The syncytiotrophoblast is a multinucleated protoplasmic mass derived from the cytotrophoblast. This layer is devoid of cell boundaries. The syncytiotrophoblast is actively involved during implantation and produces substances that cause the decidual reaction. Later, this layer produces two protein hormones and two steroid hormones.

15. **B** The amniotic cavity lies between the cytotrophoblast and the epiblast of the embryonic disc. Cells from the epiblast (amnioblasts) soon form a thin roof over this cavity called the amnion. It is continuous with the epiblast of the embryonic disc.

16. **C** The most common site of an ectopic pregnancy is the uterine tube, usually in the ampulla or isthmus. The incidence of tubal pregnancy ranges from 1 in 80 to 1 in 250 pregnancies, depending on the geographic location, socioeconomic level, and age of the pregnant woman. Pelvic inflammatory disease is a common cause of tubal ectopic pregnancy. As the embryo increases in size, the uterine tube ruptures, leading to hemorrhage and a serious threat to the mother's life.

17. **B** In an abdominal pregnancy, the conceptus develops on the peritoneal surfaces of the abdominal cavity. Abdominal pregnancies are relatively uncommon (about 0.03% of all ectopic pregnancies), and they are usually associated with intra-abdominal hemorrhage and severe abdominal pain. Rarely the embryo continues to develop until term and a live fetus may be delivered surgically. In some cases, the abdominal fetus dies and becomes calcified, forming a so-called stone fetus or lithopedion.

18. **A** The blastocyst usually implants on the superior part of the posterior wall of the uterine cavity. Implantation occurs slightly more often on the posterior than on the anterior wall.

19. **E** Implantation of the blastocyst in the uterine cervix in the region of the internal os may cover the entrance to the cervix, resulting in a condition known as placenta previa, in which the placenta may completely or partially cover the internal opening of the cervical canal. Serious hemorrhage may occur as a result of premature separation of the placenta during pregnancy or at delivery.

20. **D** Ovarian pregnancy is relatively uncommon, with an incidence of approximately 0.5% of all ectopic pregnancies. In an ovarian pregnancy, fertilization of the oocyte probably occurs in the ampulla of the uterine tube with subsequent implantation in the ovary after becoming dislodged from the tube. Because of intra-abdominal hemorrhage and other medical complications, surgical management is necessary.

# Formation of Germ Layers and Early Tissue and Organ Differentiation

## 4

## Objectives

Be able to:

- Describe the formation and growth of the primitive streak.
- Define primitive streak, primitive knot, primitive groove, and primitive pit.
- Trace the development of the notochord, using simple diagrammatic sections of 3-week embryos.
- Define notochordal process, notochordal canal, and notochordal plate.
- Give an account of the development of the neural tube, using simple sketches.
- Define neural plate, neural groove, neural folds, and neural crest.
- Illustrate, with simple sketches, the development of the following: somites, paraxial mesoderm, intermediate mesoderm, lateral mesoderm, intraembryonic coelom, tertiary villi, blood, and blood vessels.
- Construct and label diagrams showing the early development of the cardiovascular system and the sites of blood formation (blood islands).
- Write brief notes on the allantois, oropharyngeal membrane, and cloacal membrane.

## Five-Choice Completion Questions

**Directions:** Each of the following statements or questions is followed by five suggested responses or completions. **Select the one best answer** in each case.

1. Human chorionic gonadotropin (hCG) is a hormone produced by the
   - A. syncytiotrophoblast
   - B. anterior lobe of pituitary gland
   - C. corpus luteum of pregnancy
   - D. theca folliculi
   - E. hypophysis

2. The primitive streak first appears at the beginning of the _____ week.
   - A. first
   - B. second
   - C. third
   - D. fourth
   - E. fifth

3. The notochordal process lengthens by migration of cells from the
   A. notochord
   B. primitive streak
   C. notochordal plate
   D. primitive node
   E. neural plate

4. The notochordal plate infolds to form the
   A. neural tube
   B. neurenteric canal
   C. notochordal process
   D. notochordal canal
   E. notochord

5. During the third week, the neurenteric canal connects the amniotic cavity and the
   A. allantois
   B. neural tube
   C. caudal neuropore
   D. yolk sac
   E. chorionic cavity

6. The intraembryonic coelom located cranial to the oropharyngeal membrane becomes the
   A. cavity of pharynx
   B. stomodeum
   C. pericardial cavity
   D. pharyngeal cavity
   E. pleural cavity

7. The cloacal membrane consists of
   A. embryonic endoderm, mesoderm, and ectoderm
   B. a circular area of endoderm fused to embryonic mesoderm
   C. endoderm of the roof of the yolk sac and embryonic ectoderm
   D. the prechordal plate and the overlying embryonic ectoderm
   E. extraembryonic layers of the mesoderm

8. The specialized group of mesenchymal cells that aggregate to form blood islands are called
   A. hemoblasts
   B. angioblasts
   C. fibroblasts
   D. mesoblasts
   E. reticular cells

9. The primordial blood cells of the 3-week embryo first begin to form
   A. at 19 to 20 days
   B. in the embryonic disc
   C. on the yolk sac
   D. in the liver
   E. on the allantois

10. A pregnant woman who has missed two menstrual periods wants to know her expected date of delivery. In practice, which of the following would you use?
    A. menstrual history
    B. date of coitus
    C. time of ovulation
    D. probable time of fertilization
    E. vaginal examination

11. A complete hydatidiform mole was diagnosed in a 30-year-old woman with a history of intermittent bleeding during the first trimester. This disorder is associated with
    A. dispermy in most cases
    B. presence of tertiary villi
    C. decrease in hCG production
    D. nuclear DNA of maternal origin
    E. cystic swelling of chorionic villi

12. Ultrasonography revealed the presence of a sacrococcygeal teratoma in a near-term fetus. Which of the following is involved in this tumor?

A. persistence of notochord
B. primitive streak cells
C. prechordal plate

D. extraembryonic mesoderm
E. neural plate

13. During the third week of development
    A. cranial and caudal neuropores close
    B. embryonic heart can be detected
       ultrasonographically

    C. 42 to 46 pairs of somites are present
    D. secondary villi become tertiary villi
    E. embryonic disc begins to fold

14. The primitive streak
    A. extends from the primitive node
    B. is caudal to the notochord
    C. becomes the vertebral column

    D. is a thickening of endoderm
    E. induces the formation of the neural tube

15. The chromosomes of complete hydatidiform moles are
    A. always maternal in origin
    B. entirely of paternal origin
    C. always dispermic

    D. always monospermic
    E. both maternal and paternal in origin

16. Periodic segmentation of the paraxial mesoderm to form somites is controlled by the expression of
    A. noggin
    B. Sonic hedgehog (Shh)
    C. Wnt pathway

    D. notch pathway
    E. TGF-β

17. Left-right patterning of the embryonic disc is likely regulated by
    A. Sonic hedgehog
    B. nodal
    C. calcium

    D. FGFs
    E. retinoic acid

## Answers and Explanations

1. **A**  The syncytiotrophoblast produces hCG, which stimulates the corpus luteum of pregnancy to increase in size and to continue producing hormones. Progesterone produced by the corpus luteum is necessary for maintenance of pregnancy during the early months. Thereafter, progesterone is produced by the placenta.

2. **C**  The primitive streak usually appears in 15-day embryos (i.e., at the beginning of the third week). Cells from the primitive streak in the epiblast pass between the ectoderm and the endoderm and form the third germ layer (intraembryonic mesoderm).

3. **D**  If you chose **B**, the primitive streak, you are partly right because the primitive node is

the cranial end of the primitive streak. Cells migrate cranially from the primitive node to form a midline cord known as the notochordal process. The primitive node is a thickening of the epiblast at the cranial end of the primitive streak. In addition to forming the notochordal process, cells from the primitive node also form intraembryonic mesoderm.

4. **E**  The notochordal plate infolds to form the notochord. The primordium of the notochord is the notochordal process. The notochordal canal develops in the notochordal process as the primitive pit invaginates into it.

5. **D**  The neurenteric canal is associated with late stages of notochord development. It represents the part of the notochordal canal that does not

disappear when the floor of the notochordal process degenerates. The neurenteric canal connects the amniotic cavity and the yolk sac. It usually disappears when the notochord is fully developed (about 5 weeks). In most cases, the brief existence of the canal is of no significance.

6. **C**  The pericardial cavity and the developing heart are carried ventrally within the head fold as the brain grows rapidly during the fourth week. The pericardial cavity forms by confluence of isolated spaces in the cardiogenic (heart-forming) mesoderm, which lies cranial to the oropharyngeal membrane.

7. **C**  The cloacal membrane is the circular bilaminar area where the embryonic endoderm of the roof of the yolk sac contacts and fuses with the overlying embryonic ectoderm caudal to the primitive streak. There is no mesoderm between the two layers composing the cloacal membrane. The area where the prechordal plate fuses with the overlying ectoderm is the oropharyngeal membrane.

8. **B**  Angioblasts are mesenchymal cells that give rise to blood and the vascular and lymphatic systems. Fibroblasts are connective tissue cells that form fibrous tissues in the body. Hemoblasts are blood cells that usually are called hemangioblasts. Reticular cells and fibers form a network surrounding the blood islands and sinusoids.

9. **C**  Primordial blood first forms in the extraembryonic mesoderm on the yolk sac at 15 to 16 days. Later it forms in the allantois and connecting stalk. Blood formation does not begin in the embryo until the sixth week, when it forms in the liver. Hemopoiesis begins in the spleen during the second trimester and in bone marrow before the beginning of the third trimester. Homeobox genes, growth factors, and cytokines play an essential role in regulating blood cell formation. Hence, the blood in the 3-week embryo forms in the extraembryonic membranes and flows into the cardiovascular system as the embryonic vessels form.

10. **A**  In practice, the age of the embryo is calculated from the first day of the last normal menstrual period (LNMP) because this information usually is readily available. The most accurate estimation of the date of delivery is from the time of fertilization because the oocyte usually is fertilized within 12 hours after ovulation. Clinical signs of pregnancy may be evident by vaginal examination by about the sixth week because of an increase in uterine size and softening of the cervix. The fundus of the uterus can be palpated from the abdominal wall by the third month. Ultrasonography is commonly used for estimating embryonic and fetal age.

11. **E**  A hydatidiform mole results from abnormal proliferation of the trophoblast even though the embryo is dead. The chorionic villi do not become vascularized to form tertiary villi and soon degenerate to form a large mass of cystic swellings. The excessive trophoblast produces large amounts of hCG. About 2% of these moles develop into malignant lesions called choriocarcinomas, which typically metastasize to various parts of the body (e.g., the lungs, liver, vagina, and brain). The nuclear DNA is paternal in origin. More than 90% of complete hydatidiform moles are monospermic, resulting from the fertilization of an empty oocyte by a sperm.

12. **B**  The primitive streak forms intraembryonic mesoderm until the end of the fourth week, after which it slowly regresses and disappears. Persistence of primitive streak cells gives rise to a tumor known as a teratoma in the region of the sacrum and coccyx. These tumors are more common in females than in males and may become cancerous during infancy. Because of the pleuripotent nature of primitive streak cells, many tumors contain different types of tissue.

13. **D**  By the end of the third week, blood vessels develop from mesenchymal tissue in the core of the secondary chorionic villi, transforming them into tertiary villi. By the end of the third week, the primitive heart is beating but this cannot be detected ultrasonographically until the fifth week. Somites begin to form before the end of the third week, and 42 to 44 pairs of somites are present by the end of the fifth week. The notochord induces neural tube formation during the third week, and neural

tube formation is completed during the fourth week. Folding of the embryonic disc occurs at the beginning of the fourth week.

14. **B**   The primitive streak is located caudal to the notochord, which is involved in the induction of the neural tube. The primitive streak appears at the beginning of the third week and contributes to the formation of intraembryonic mesoderm and the notochord. By the beginning of the fifth week, the primitive streak degenerates and normally disappears.

15. **B**   On the basis of karyotype and other characteristic histopathologic features, hydatidiform moles are classified as either complete or partial. The chromosomes of complete hydatidiform moles are entirely of paternal origin. More than 90% of complete hydatidiform moles are monospermic, resulting from the fertilization of an empty oocyte by a haploid sperm followed by duplication. A dispermic mole results from the fertilization of an empty oocyte by two sperms. The risk of a complete or partial mole increases after spontaneous abortion, and in some cases a molar pregnancy may lead to a trophoblastic tumor, that is, a choriocarcinoma.

16. **D**   The notch pathway of signal transduction appears to play an essential role in the periodic segmentation of the paraxial mesoderm to form somites, a process known as somitogenesis. TGF-$\beta$ factors are involved in mesoderm formation. Hox genes, noggin, Wnt, and Shh are involved in the patterning of the somites.

17. **B**   Nodal, a TGF-$\beta$ related protein, is first expressed at the primitive node of the primitive streak. Experimental studies show that nodal plays an essential role in the differentiation and migration of mesenchymal cells (gastrulation) to form intraembryonic mesoderm, as well as right-left axis of the embryonic disc.

# *Five-Choice Association Questions*

**Directions:** Each group of questions below consists of a numbered list of descriptive words or phrases accompanied by a diagram with certain parts indicated by letters and a list of lettered headings. For each numbered word or phrase, **select the lettered part or heading** that matches it correctly and then insert the letter in the space to the right of the appropriate number. Sometimes more than one numbered word or phrase may be correctly matched to the same lettered part or heading.

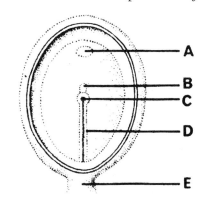

A. Allantois
B. Primitive streak
C. Notochord
D. Blood island
E. Neural plate

1. _____ Notochordal process
2. _____ Site of prechordal plate
3. _____ Gives rise to most of embryonic mesoderm
4. _____ Ventral layer of oropharyngeal membrane
5. _____ Primitive pit

6. _____ Aggregation of angioblasts
7. _____ Diverticulum of yolk sac
8. _____ Induces embryonic ectoderm to thicken
9. _____ Forms basis of axial skeleton
10. _____ Gives rise to brain and spinal cord
11. _____ Source of mesenchyme
12. _____ Rudimentary structure
13. _____ Appears on extraembryonic membranes

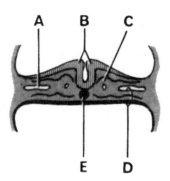

14. _____ Wall of amniotic sac
15. _____ Neural groove
16. _____ Derived from primitive streak
17. _____ Embryonic ectoderm

18. _____ Derived from paraxial mesoderm
19. _____ Derived from notochordal process
20. _____ Gives rise to an adult body cavity
21. _____ Splanchnopleure
22. _____ Fusing to form neural tube

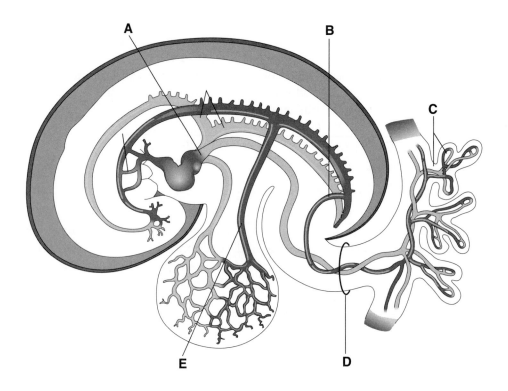

23. _____ Umbilical artery
24. _____ Vitelline artery
25. _____ Sinus venosus

26. _____ Contains umbilical vessels
27. _____ Tertiary chorionic villus

---

## Answers and Explanations

1. **B** The notochordal process is a rod-shaped structure composed of cells derived from the primitive node of the primitive streak. It is the primordium of the notochord, a cellular structure that defines the primordial axis of the embryo.

2. **A** The site of the prechordal plate is indicated in the drawing by a dotted oval to indicate that it is not visible from the dorsal surface of the embryonic disc. The prechordal plate is a circular area of thickened embryonic endoderm in the cranial part of the roof of the yolk sac.

The prechordal plate, together with the overlying embryonic ectoderm, later constitutes the oropharyngeal membrane.

3. **D**   The primitive streak, a linear band of epiblast, gives rise to mesoderm mainly during the third week. The mesoderm extends laterally and becomes continuous with the extraembryonic mesoderm on the amnion and yolk sac.

4. **A**   The ventral layer of the bilaminar oropharyngeal membrane is the prechordal plate; the dorsal layer is embryonic ectoderm. This membrane ruptures during the fourth week, bringing the primordial oral cavity into communication with the primordial pharynx.

5. **C**   The primitive pit is a depression in the primitive node at the cranial end of the primitive streak. It extends into the notochordal process and forms the notochordal canal. Thus, it is the entrance to the notochordal canal. The pit later forms the opening of the neurenteric canal, which temporarily connects the amniotic cavity with the yolk sac.

6. **D**   Splanchnic mesenchymal cells known as angioblasts aggregate to form isolated masses called blood islands, which develop into vascular endothelium and primordial blood cells. Blood islands form first on the yolk sac, chorion, allantois, and connecting stalk, but they develop in the embryo about 2 days later.

7. **A**   The allantois, a diverticulum of the yolk sac, is a vestigial structure that later becomes the urachus (median umbilical ligament in an adult). It serves as a reservoir for excretory products in some species, but it is nonfunctional in human embryos. However, its blood vessels become the umbilical vessels.

8. **C**   The developing notochord and the adjacent paraxial mesoderm are thought to produce inductive substances that stimulate development of the neural plate from the overlying embryonic ectoderm.

9. **C**   The notochord forms the basis of the axial skeleton. The vertebrae develop around it, and then it degenerates. In between the vertebrae,

the notochord forms the primordium of the nucleus pulposus of the intervertebral disc.

10. **E**   The neural plate is a thickened area of ectoderm that overlies and extends on each side of the notochord. The neural plate invaginates to form a neural groove. In later development, the neural folds meet dorsally and fuse to form the neural tube. The cranial part of the neural tube develops into the brain, and the longer remaining part forms the spinal cord. The notochord and paraxial mesoderm produce inductive substances that stimulate or induce the overlying ectoderm to thicken and form the neural plate.

11. **B**   The primitive streak produces mesoderm, which develops into mesenchyme (embryonic connective tissue). Mesenchyme forms a packing tissue around developing organs and develops into connective tissues and muscles.

12. **A**   The allantois is a rudimentary structure. Although the allantois does not function in human embryos, it is important because blood formation occurs in its walls and its blood vessels become the umbilical vessels.

13. **D**   The blood islands first appear on the walls of the yolk sac, allantois, and connecting stalk. These extraembryonic membranes are derived from the zygote, but they are not part of the embryo. Blood islands form in the embryo about 2 days after they appear on the yolk sac.

14. **C**   The amnion encloses the amniotic cavity, forming an amniotic sac. It contains fluid that bathes the embryonic disc, forming its floor. The wall of this sac consists of an inner epithelial layer of cells covered externally by extraembryonic somatic mesoderm.

15. **A**   The neural groove forms as the neural plate invaginates to form a neural fold on each side. The folds later fuse to form the neural tube, the primordium of the central nervous system (brain and spinal cord). The ectoderm lateral to the folds, surface ectoderm, gives rise to the epidermis of the skin.

16. **E**   The intraembryonic mesoderm is derived from the primitive streak. The primitive streak

produces mesoderm rapidly during the third and fourth weeks.

17. **B**   The embryonic ectoderm in the region indicated forms a neural fold. The neural folds soon fuse, converting the neural plate into the neural tube.

18. **C**   The somites are paired cubical masses derived by segmentation of the paraxial mesoderm. The first pair of somites is formed a short distance caudal to the tip of the notochord, and successive somites are progressively formed from paraxial mesoderm. Most somites appear between days 20 and 30; they give rise to the axial skeleton and its associated musculature.

19. **E**   The notochord arises by transformation of the notochordal process. The notochord is a cellular rod that defines the primordial axis of the embryo. Mesenchymal cells from the somites later surround it and give rise to the mesenchymal bodies of the vertebrae. The notochord within the developing vertebrae later degenerates.

20. **A**   The intraembryonic coelom in the area indicated becomes part of the peritoneal cavity. The coelom appears here as a space within the lateral mesoderm, splitting it into somatic and splanchnic layers. The transverse section is cut through the caudal region of the lateral extensions of the horseshoe-shaped body cavity or coelom.

21. **D**   The splanchnopleure is composed of splanchnic mesoderm and endoderm and represents the future wall of the primordial gut. The endoderm gives rise to the epithelium and glands of the digestive tract, and the mesoderm gives rise to its muscular and fibrous elements.

22. **B**   The neural folds are fusing to form the neural tube, the primordium of the brain and spinal cord. These folds form as the neural plate invaginates along its central axis to form a neural groove.

23. **B**   The paired umbilical arteries are branches of the dorsal aortae. They transport deoxygenated blood and waste products from the embryo to the chorionic villi of the placenta.

24. **E**   The vitelline arteries are branches of the dorsal aortae to the yolk sac. The vitelline arteries and vitelline veins are in communication through the vascular plexus on the yolk sac.

25. **A**   Blood enters the sinus venosus from the embryo through the cardinal veins, from the developing placenta via the umbilical vein, and from the yolk sac via the vitelline veins. Blood from the sinus venosus enters the primordial heart.

26. **D**   The umbilical cord develops from the connecting stalk. It contains the paired umbilical arteries and the umbilical vein. The umbilical cord is the vital connection between the embryo and the placenta because the umbilical vessels transport gases (e.g., oxygen), nutrients, essential substances, and waste products.

27. **C**   By the end of the third week, blood vessels differentiate from mesenchymal cells in the core of the secondary villi to form the tertiary chorionic villi. The blood vessels in these villi soon become connected with the primordial heart via blood vessels that differentiate in the mesenchyme of the chorion and connecting stalk. A primordial embryonic circulation is established by the end of the third week. Oxygen and nutrients in the maternal blood in the intervillous spaces diffuse through the walls of the villi and enter the embryo's blood. Carbon dioxide and waste products diffuse from fetal blood through the walls of the villi into the maternal blood.

# Organogenetic Period: The Fourth to Eighth Weeks

**5**

## Objectives

Be able to:

- Explain why the fourth to eighth weeks are a critical period of human development.
- Define neuropore, pharyngeal arch, aortic arch, otic pit, lens placode, limb bud, and cervical flexure.
- Estimate the age of embryos previously traced from drawings, using the table in your textbook and crown-rump measurements.
- Briefly indicate what each germ layer normally contributes to the tissues and organs of the embryo.
- Discuss induction, using the eye as an example.
- Discuss the establishment of general body form resulting from folding of the embryo, with special reference to the effect of this process on the septum transversum, heart, foregut, midgut, allantois, and yolk sac.

## Five-Choice Completion Questions

**Directions:** Each of the following statements or questions is followed by five suggested responses or completions. **Select the one best answer** in each case.

1. All the essential features of external body form of the embryo are completed by the end of the _____ week.
   - A. fourth
   - B. sixth
   - C. eighth
   - D. tenth
   - E. twelfth

2. During the early part of the fourth week, the rate of growth at the periphery of the embryonic disc fails to keep pace with the rate of growth of the
   - A. yolk sac
   - B. amniotic cavity
   - C. embryonic coelom
   - D. notochordal process
   - E. neural tube

3. By the middle of the fourth week, the neural folds at the cranial end of the embryo have begun to develop into the
   - A. neural crest
   - B. spinal cord
   - C. brain
   - D. neural groove
   - E. neural tube

4. After folding of the head region, the mesodermal structure just caudal to the pericardial cavity is the
   - A. primordial heart
   - B. connecting stalk
   - C. primitive streak
   - D. septum transversum
   - E. notochord

5. Each of the following structures turns onto the ventral surface of the embryo during folding of the head, **except** the
   - A. oropharyngeal membrane
   - B. notochord
   - C. heart
   - D. pericardial cavity
   - E. septum transversum

6. The terminal dilated part of the hindgut is the:
   - A. allantois
   - B. yolk stalk
   - C. cloaca
   - D. vitelline duct
   - E. cecum

7. Each of the following structures is derived from mesoderm, **except**:
   - A. muscle
   - B. cartilage
   - C. mesenchyme
   - D. blood vessels
   - E. epidermis

8. Which of the following structures is believed to be a primary inductor during organogenesis?
   - A. somite
   - B. notochord
   - C. yolk sac
   - D. primitive streak
   - E. lens

9. Each of the following is a distinctive characteristic of a 4-week embryo, **except**:
   - A. somites
   - B. hand plates
   - C. pharyngeal arches
   - D. lower limb buds
   - E. neuropores

10. The most frequently used method for measuring the length of a 5-week embryo is
    - A. greatest length
    - B. standing height
    - C. crown-rump length
    - D. crown-heel length
    - E. total length

11. The age of the embryo illustrated below is _____ weeks.

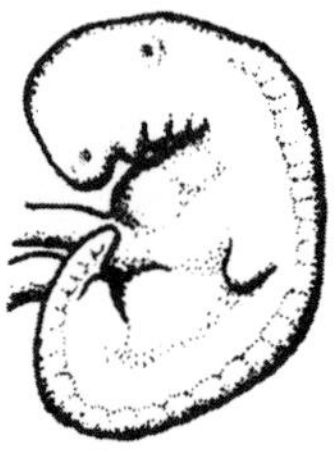

   - A. 3
   - B. 4
   - C. 5
   - D. 6
   - E. 7

12. A pathologic examination of an aborted embryo revealed that it was about 20 mm in length, with the midgut herniated into the proximal part of the umbilical cord. The trunk of the embryo was elongated and straightened. Nipples were present, and the cerebral vesicles were prominent. Digital rays of the hand and foot plates were also evident. Which of the following is likely to be the approximate age of the embryo?

A. 4 weeks  
B. 5 weeks  
C. 6 weeks  

D. 7 weeks  
E. 8 weeks  

13. Characteristics of embryos early in the eighth week include

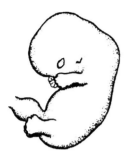

A. webbed fingers  
B. eyelids  
C. umbilical herniation  
D. tail-like caudal eminence  
E. all of the above  

14. Each of the following structures is derived from the neural crest **except**:

A. pigment cells  
B. bulbar ridges in the heart  
C. pineal body  

D. pharyngeal arch cartilages  
E. medulla of suprarenal gland  

## Answers and Explanations

1. **C** By the end of the embryonic period (8 weeks), the beginnings of all major external and internal structures have developed. Therefore, these 5 weeks constitute the most critical period of development and the time when major developmental anomalies may occur.

2. **E** Because of the rapid growth of the neural tube, the embryo bulges into the amniotic cavity and the head and tail regions fold under the cranial and caudal parts of the embryonic disc. Concurrently, marked folding occurs along the lateral margins of the disc.

3. **C** By the middle of the fourth week, the neural folds at the center of the embryo have started to move together and fuse into the neural tube. At the cranial end of the embryo, the thick neural folds indicate where the brain will develop. By the end of the fourth week, the neural folds in the cranial region have fused to form primary brain vesicles, which develop into the brain.

4. **D** The mesodermal mass — septum transversum — forms the caudal wall of the pericardial cavity. This transverse mesodermal septum is the primordium of the central tendon of the diaphragm. After folding of the head, the heart

lies dorsal to the pericardial cavity. The primitive streak and connecting stalk lie considerably caudal to the pericardial cavity.

5. **B** The cranial end of the notochord may bend slightly as the forebrain folds ventrally, but the notochord does not turn onto the ventral surface as the other structures do (e.g., the heart).

6. **C** Shortly after the caudal part of the yolk sac is incorporated into the embryo as the hindgut, the terminal part of the hindgut dilates to form the cloaca. Its cavity is separated from the amniotic cavity by the cloacal membrane.

7. **E** The epidermis is derived from surface ectoderm. The dermis of the skin is derived from mesoderm, as are all types of connective tissue. The cartilages in the pharyngeal arches are derived from neural crest cells.

8. **B** Substances produced by the notochordal process and later the notochord induce the neural plate to form. The lenses function as secondary inductors.

9. **B** Upper limb buds are present but hand plates are not visible until the fifth week. They

are not distinctive characteristics of the limbs until the fifth week.

10. **C**   Crown-rump measurements are most commonly taken. Greatest length is used for a straight embryo (e.g., during the third week). Crown-heel measurements (standing height) are sometimes used for an older embryo, but they often are difficult to make on a formalin-fixed embryo because it is difficult to straighten. Ultrasound measurements are used to determine the age of an embryo in utero.

11. **B**   The distinctive characteristics of the 4-week embryo shown here are: four pharyngeal arches, a flipper-like upper limb bud, and a small lower limb bud.

12. **D**   The embryo is about 7 weeks. Umbilical herniation is usually obvious during this period. Before the seventh week, the embryo is somewhat curved and has hand and foot plates. After the seventh week, notches appear between the digital rays and the digits are formed. By the seventh week, the nipples and the prominent cerebral vesicles are evident.

13. **E**   Webbed fingers and notches between the digits of the feet are characteristic features of embryos during the early part of the eighth week. The presence of eyelids, a short tail-like caudal eminence, and the umbilical herniation are also features of the early part of this week.

14. **C**   Neuroectodermal cells become segregated to form the neural crest following fusion of the neural folds and formation of the neural tube. The pineal body is derived from the neural tube (brain). Pigment cells, the medulla of the suprarenal gland, pharyngeal arch cartilages, bulbar ridges in the heart, as well as other structures, develop from neural crest cells.

## *Five-Choice Association Questions*

**Directions:** Each group of questions below consists of a numbered list of descriptive words or phrases accompanied by a diagram with certain parts indicated by letters or by a list of lettered headings. For each numbered word or phrase, **select the letter or heading** that matches it correctly. Then insert the letter in the space to the right of the appropriate number. Sometimes more than one numbered word or phrase may be correctly matched to the same lettered part or heading.

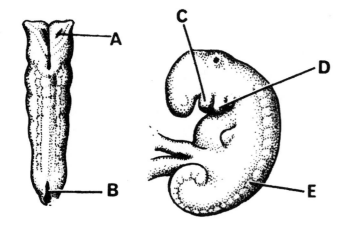

1. _____ Hyoid arch
2. _____ Gives rise to mandible
3. _____ Forms from paraxial mesoderm
4. _____ First pharyngeal arch
5. _____ Neuropore
6. _____ Optic groove in neural fold

7. _____ Forms major part of diaphragm
8. _____ Primordial mouth
9. _____ Outgrowth of ventrolateral body wall
10. _____ Forms as a result of head fold
11. _____ Closes during fourth week
12. _____ Ectodermal depression in neck

A. Limb bud
B. Neuropore
C. Septum transversum
D. Cervical sinus
E. Stomodeum

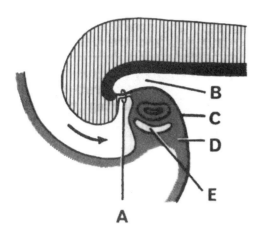

A. fourth week
B. fifth week
C. sixth week
D. seventh week
E. eighth week

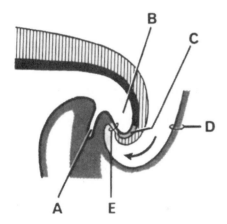

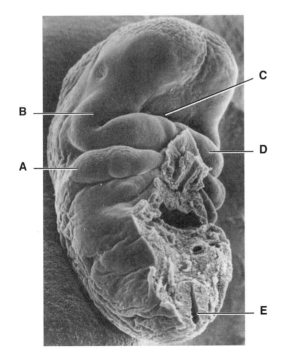

13. _____ Septum transversum
14. _____ Part of embryonic coelom
15. _____ Oropharyngeal membrane
16. _____ Separates amniotic cavity from foregut
17. _____ Gives rise to a major part of diaphragm

18. _____ Lens placodes recognizable
19. _____ Umbilical herniation noticeable
20. _____ Retinal pigment first recognizable
21. _____ Lower limb buds appear
22. _____ Embryo essentially straight
23. _____ Cervical sinuses visible
24. _____ Caudal eminence (tailbud) disappears

25. _____ Cloaca
26. _____ Produces embryonic mesoderm
27. _____ Separates amniotic cavity from hindgut
28. _____ Vestigial structure
29. _____ Amnion
30. _____ Site of blood formation in early embryo

31. _____ Second pharyngeal arch
32. _____ Derived from neural tube
33. _____ Stomodeum
34. _____ Will form lower jaw
35. _____ Gives rise to upper jaw
36. _____ Defect in its formation results in a
    severe type of spina bifida

## Answers and Explanations

1. **D**  The second or hyoid pharyngeal arch is recognizable early in the fourth week. As its name implies, this arch gives rise to part of the hyoid bone. Mesenchyme in this arch also gives rise to the muscles of facial expression and to various skeletal structures.

2. **C**  The mandibular prominences of the first pair of pharyngeal arches give rise to the lower jaw or mandible. Rostral extensions of the first arch — maxillary prominences — give rise to the upper jaw or maxilla.

3. **E**  The somites form by differentiation and division of longitudinal columns of paraxial mesoderm into cubical segments. The somites give rise to most of the axial skeleton, the associated musculature, and the dermis of the skin.

4. **C**  The pointer indicates the mandibular prominence of the first pharyngeal arch. The mandibular prominences merge with each other during the fourth week and give rise to the mandible, lower lip, and inferior part of the face.

5. **B**  The caudal neuropore is indicated. The neuropores (rostral and caudal) normally close by the end of the fourth week. The rostral neuropore closes on day 25 or 26, and the caudal neuropore usually closes about 2 days later. Defective closure of the caudal neuropore gives rise to a severe anomaly — spina bifida.

6. **A**  The pointer indicates the optic groove in a neural fold. This sulcus is the primordium of the optic vesicle, an outgrowth of the forebrain vesicle.

7. **C**  The septum transversum is a mass of mesoderm that appears cranial to the developing heart. After folding of the embryo, it lies caudal to the heart, where it forms part of the primordial diaphragm. Later it develops into the central tendon of the diaphragm.

8. **E**  The stomodeum or primordial mouth is an ectodermal depression that develops during the fourth week as the head folds. Initially, it is separated from the primordial pharynx (cranial part of foregut) by the oropharyngeal membrane. By the end of the fourth week, this membrane ruptures, bringing the mouth into communication with the foregut.

9. **A**  The limb buds form on the ventrolateral body wall during the fourth week. The upper limb buds usually appear on day 26, and the lower limb buds are visible about 2 days later.

10. **E**  The stomodeum and foregut form as the head folds ventrally. The cranial part of the yolk sac is incorporated into the embryo during this longitudinal folding. At first, the stomodeum and foregut are separate cavities, but they become continuous during the fourth week when the oropharyngeal membrane ruptures.

11. **B**  The neuropores close during the fourth week. The rostral neuropore closes on day 25 or 26, and the caudal neuropore closes about 2 days later. Defects of closure of the neuropores give rise to congenital anomalies of the central nervous system (e.g., spina bifida).

12. **D**  The cervical sinus is a depression in the surface ectoderm on each side of the future neck. It forms when the second pharyngeal arch overgrows the third and fourth arches. The second and third arches come to lie at the bottom of a pit — the cervical sinus. It is visible externally only during the fifth week.

13. **D**  The septum transversum is a mass of mesoderm that is first recognizable cranial to the pericardial coelom. After folding, it lies caudal to the heart and pericardial coelom. The septum transversum gives rise to the central tendon of the definitive diaphragm.

14. **E**  The pericardial coelom is the part of the embryonic coelom that gives rise to the pericardial cavity. It first appears in the cardiogenic mesoderm, where it lies cranial to the oropharyngeal membrane. After folding, the pericardial coelom lies ventral to the developing heart, as shown in the drawing.

15. **A** The oropharyngeal membrane develops during the third week as the prechordal plate fuses with the overlying embryonic ectoderm. This membrane ruptures during the fourth week.

16. **A** The oropharyngeal membrane separates the amniotic cavity from the foregut. Amniotic fluid may enter the primordial mouth or stomodeum, but it cannot pass into the primordial pharynx until the oropharyngeal membrane ruptures.

17. **D** The septum transversum is the first recognizable part of the developing diaphragm. It appears cranially at the end of the third week, when the pericardial coelom forms. The septum transversum later forms the central tendon of the diaphragm.

18. **A** Lens placodes are recognizable during the fourth week as thickenings of the surface ectoderm. They give rise to the lens vesicles, the primordia of the lenses of the eyes.

19. **D** As the midgut loop develops, it herniates into the umbilical cord because there is not enough room for it in the abdomen. This physiologic process or herniation begins during the fifth week, but the intestines do not usually form a noticeable swelling of the cord until the seventh week.

20. **B** Pigment appears in the retina of the eye during the fifth week, making the eyes more obvious. Eye development is first evident early in the fourth week, when the optic grooves develop.

21. **A** Lower limb buds appear toward the end of the fourth week as ventrolateral swellings of the body walls. Each bud consists of a mass of mesenchyme that is covered by surface ectoderm. The upper limb buds form around the middle of the fourth week.

22. **A** The embryo is essentially straight during the early part of the fourth week. Near the middle of the fourth week, the embryo begins to fold in the longitudinal and horizontal planes, giving the embryo a C-shaped curvature.

23. **B** Cervical sinuses are visible externally during the fifth week. The external openings of these sinuses usually close by the end of the fifth week. Remnants of parts of the cervical sinuses may give rise to anomalies — lateral cervical cysts.

24. **E** The caudal eminence is visible during the early part of the eighth week, but it disappears by the end of the eighth week.

25. **B** The cloaca is the dilated caudal part of the hindgut; the allantois enters it ventrally. The cloaca is separated from the amniotic cavity by the cloacal membrane.

26. **C** The primitive streak appears during the early part of the third week and produces mesoderm rapidly until the end of the fourth week. Thereafter, mesoderm production from this source slows down.

27. **E** The cloacal membrane separates the amniotic cavity from the cloacal region of the hindgut. This membrane consists of fused layers of embryonic ectoderm and endoderm. It is later divided into anal and urogenital membranes during the seventh week; these membranes soon rupture.

28. **A** The allantois is a vestigial structure that forms during the third week as a diverticulum of the caudal wall of the yolk sac. It remains very small and gives rise to the urachus, a tubular structure that runs from the urinary bladder to the umbilicus. Its adult derivative is the median umbilical ligament.

29. **D** The amnion forms during the second week. It is attached to the margins of the embryonic disc and forms the wall of the amniotic sac.

30. **A** Blood begins to form in the mesenchyme around the allantois and yolk sac during the third week. These are the only sites of blood formation until blood begins to form in the liver during the sixth week.

31. **A** The second pharyngeal arch appears at the beginning of the fourth week. The embryo is about 32 days' after fertilization with four pairs

of pharyngeal arches; the fourth pharyngeal arch is smaller and not clearly delineated. The second pharyngeal arch overgrows the third and fourth arches, forming a transitory ectoderm-lined cervical sinus that becomes obliterated.

32. **E**   The neural tube is formed following fusion of the neural folds by the end of the fourth week. It gives rise to the brain and spinal cord.

33. **C**   An ectoderm-lined depression — the stomodeum — partly contributes to the formation of the oral cavity. It is located at the cranial end of the embryo, bounded by the maxillary and mandibular prominences. The oropharyngeal membrane breaks down at about 26 days, bringing the primordial pharynx into communication with the amniotic cavity.

34. **D**   The first pharyngeal arch gives rise to both the maxillary and mandibular prominences.

The lower jaw is formed from the larger mandibular prominences, which are paired at first, but the medial ends merge and fuse during the fourth week.

35. **B**   The shorter and smaller maxillary prominences form the lateral boundaries of the stomodeum. The maxillary prominences, which lie just below the overhanging frontonasal prominence, grow medially and merge with the medial nasal prominences to form the upper lip. The upper jaw develops from the maxillary prominences, which also give rise to several facial and cranial bones.

36. **E**   Fusion of the neural folds occurs during the fourth week, forming the neural tube. The neural tube gives rise to the brain and spinal cord. Neural tube defects, including a severe type of spina bifida, occur as a result of defective closure of the neural tube.

# Fetal Period

**6**

## Objectives

Be able to:

- State the significant differences between development during the embryonic and fetal periods, and comment on differences in the vulnerability of embryos and fetuses to teratogenic agents.

- Discuss the effects of an inadequate uterine environment, indicating the possible effects of environmental agents (e.g., viruses) and other factors on fetal growth and development.

- Describe the differences between fetuses that are of low birth weight because of intrauterine growth retardation (IUGR) and those that are premature.

- Write brief notes on the following techniques used for assessing the status of the human fetus before birth: amniocentesis, fetal blood sampling, chorionic villus sampling, and ultrasonography.

## Five-Choice Completion Questions

**Directions:** Each of the following statements or questions is followed by five suggested responses or completions. **Select the one best answer** in each case.

1. The head constitutes almost half the fetus at the beginning of the
   - A. 12th week
   - B. second trimester
   - C. fetal period
   - D. stage of quickening
   - E. embryonic period

2. The usual measurement for estimating fetal age is
   - A. crown-rump length
   - B. foot length
   - C. crown-heel length
   - D. leg length
   - E. head size

3. Which of the following statements about fetal age and weight is closest to the normal relationship?
   - A. 8 weeks — 10 gm
   - B. 12 weeks — 200 gm
   - C. 20 weeks — 800 gm
   - D. 26 weeks — 1000 gm
   - E. 38 weeks — 4400 gm

4. The fetal period begins
   - A. after all organs have completely developed
   - B. when the genitalia have distinctive characteristics
   - C. at the beginning of the ninth week
   - D. at the end of the first trimester
   - E. when the fetus is viable

5. Sexing of fetuses is possible from examination of the external genitalia during the _____ week.
   A. eighth
   B. ninth
   C. tenth
   D. eleventh
   E. twelfth

6. A fetus has a reasonable chance of surviving, if born prematurely, when its fertilization age is _____ weeks.
   A. 12
   B. 16
   C. 18
   D. 20
   E. 24

7. Quickening, the period when fetal movements commonly are felt by the mother, usually occurs
   A. near the end of the first trimester
   B. around the middle of the second trimester
   C. at the end of the second trimester
   D. when the fetus becomes viable
   E. during the so-called finishing period

8. The most likely cause of very low birth weight in a full-term fetus is
   A. maternal malnutrition
   B. prematurity
   C. smoking
   D. placental insufficiency
   E. alcoholism

9. Amniocentesis is commonly used to
   A. diagnose the chromosomal sex of fetuses
   B. detect placental insufficiency
   C. assess the degree of erythroblastosis fetalis
   D. determine the composition of the amniotic fluid
   E. determine the age of the fetus

10. Which of the following ultrasonographic measurements is most reliable for estimating fetal age during the first trimester?
   A. crown-rump length (CRL)
   B. diameter of the head
   C. dimension of the trunk
   D. foot length
   E. cheek to cheek

11. The age of a fetus was estimated from measurements of its CRL using ultrasonography. How early can the sex of the fetus be clearly determined from the appearance of its external genitalia?
   A. 9 weeks
   B. 10 weeks
   C. 12 weeks
   D. 14 weeks
   E. 16 weeks

12. Primary ossification centers appear in the long bones of a fetus at
   A. 9 weeks
   B. 13 weeks
   C. 17 weeks
   D. 21 weeks
   E. 25 weeks

13. A woman who is 8 weeks pregnant asked her doctor when she should feel her "baby" moving. The reply should be, at about
   A. 10 weeks
   B. 12 weeks
   C. 17 weeks
   D. 22 weeks
   E. 30 weeks

14. Oligohydramnios was diagnosed in a pregnant woman. This condition is associated with
    A. increased amniotic fluid volume
    D. esophageal atresia
    B. meroanencephaly (anencephaly)
    E. twin pregnancy
    C. fetal renal disease

15. In a pregnancy that was medically terminated, a nonviable male fetus was recovered. The fetus had a CRL of 160 mm. The skin was covered with vernix caseosa. Fingernails and toenails were not present, and the eyelids were closed. This fetus is probably about _____ weeks old.
    A. 14                          D. 28
    B. 18                          E. 32
    C. 22

16. An infant born after a prolonged pregnancy showed signs of the postmaturity syndrome, which includes the following characteristic feature
    A. low birth weight            D. abundant lanugo
    B. dry parchment-like skin     E. short fingernails
    C. increased vernix caseosa + 13

---

## Answers and Explanations

1. **C** At 9 weeks, when the fetal period begins, the head constitutes almost one-half of the fetus. Thereafter, growth of the head slows down compared with the rest of the body. By the end of the 12th week, the head represents almost one-third of the length of the fetus. The stage of quickening, or the time when the fetal movements are recognized by the mother, does not occur until the 17- to 20-week period. By this stage, the head represents a little more than one-fourth of the length of the fetus.

2. **A** Crown-rump measurements are the most useful criteria for estimating fetal age. The crown rump length (CRL) of fetuses, like those of infants, varies considerably for a given age. Crown-heel measurements often are used for older fetuses, but they are less useful because of the difficulty in straightening the fetus. Foot length correlates well with CRL and is particularly useful for estimating the age of incomplete or macerated fetuses. Head size is used to estimate the age of mature fetuses (e.g., after 22 weeks).

3. **D** Most fetuses of 26 weeks weigh about 1000 gm and survive if born prematurely. Al-though there is no sharp limit of development, age, or weight at which a fetus becomes viable, most fetuses that are younger than 22 weeks or weigh less than 500 gm do not survive. All the other weights listed are high for the ages given. For example, 8-week fetuses usually weigh about 5 gm. Full-term fetuses (38 weeks after fertilization) may weigh 4400 gm, but this is heavy. The average weight of newborn infants in North America is 3400 gm. There is an increased frequency of low birth weights among teenage mothers, largely because they are still growing and have greater nutritional requirements than do older women (i.e., young mothers compete with their fetuses for nutrients).

4. **C** The fetal period begins at the beginning of the ninth week (i.e., during the first trimester). Most organs have not completed their development when the fetal period begins. The external genitalia do not acquire distinctive sexual characteristics until the end of the ninth week, and their mature form is not established until the twelfth week. The intestines do not enter the abdomen until the 10th week, about 1 week after the beginning of the fetal period.

5. **E** The external genitalia of male and female fetuses appear somewhat similar until the end of the twelfth week. The external genitalia are fully formed at this time.

6. **E** Fetuses that weigh less than 1000 gm and are less than 24 weeks of age do not usually survive if born prematurely because of the immaturity of their respiratory systems. By 26 to 28 weeks, sufficient terminal air sacs, surfactant, and vascularity have formed for adequate gas exchange and maintenance of life.

7. **B** Fetal movements usually are felt by the mother around the middle of the second trimester of pregnancy (17 to 20 weeks). Mothers who have been pregnant three or more times (multigravida) usually feel the fetus move sooner (quickening) than mothers who are pregnant for the first time (primigravida). The fetus begins to move before the end of the first trimester, but these movements are too slight to be detected by the mother.

8. **D** Placental insufficiency, caused by placental defects (e.g., infarction or nonfunctional areas of the placenta) that reduce the area for passing nutrients to the embryo, produces the placental dysfunction syndrome. Impaired uterine blood flow, caused by severe hypotension and renal disease, can result in a slow passage of nutrients to the embryo. Severe maternal malnutrition resulting from a restricted diet of poor quality may cause low birth weight, especially in teenage mothers. Fetuses of mothers who smoke heavily usually weigh less than fetuses of nonsmokers. Prematurity is a common cause of low birth weight, but full-term fetuses cannot be premature.

9. **C** Withdrawal of samples of amniotic fluid (amniocentesis) is a major tool in assessing the degree of erythroblastosis fetalis (hemolytic disease of the fetus). This condition results from destruction of red blood cells by maternal antibodies. Some severely ill fetuses can be saved by giving them intrauterine blood transfusions. Amniotic fluid is also commonly studied to detect chromosomal abnormalities.

10. **A** Ultrasonographic crown-rump length (CRL) measurements are predictive of fetal age with an accuracy of $\pm$ 1 to 2 days. The other measurements are also useful for estimating fetal age and size but are less reliable individually. Assessment of fetal age is enhanced when the crown-rump measurements are combined with one or more of these fetal measurements.

11. **C** The early development of the external genitalia in both sexes is similar. From the ninth week, the external genitalia passes through an undifferentiated (indifferent) stage; however, by the twelfth week, distinguishing sexual characteristics are established and a male fetus can be differentiated from a female.

12. **A** Primary ossification centers are visible in the long bones at nine weeks. By the end of the twelfth week, primary ossification centers are present in the fetal skeleton, especially in the cranium and long bones. Ossification is intense between 13 and 16 weeks, and by the beginning of the sixteenth week the bones are clearly visible on sonograms taken of the mother's abdomen.

13. **C** Fetal movements — quickening — are commonly felt by the mother between 17 and 20 weeks. Prior to this period, growth of the fetus is rapid, and by the end of 20 weeks the fetus has a CRL of about 190 mm. Fetal movement is an important physiological activity for normal intrauterine development. It also indicates that the fetus is alive. Spontaneous fetal movements can be observed using sonography.

14. **C** The volume of amniotic fluid increases slowly during pregnancy, reaching a peak volume of 1000 ml between 36 and 37 weeks. In about 4% of pregnancies, the volume of amniotic fluid is markedly reduced, leading to oligohydramnios. Fetal urine contribution to the amniotic fluid decreases in cases of renal agenesis. Fetal urinary tract obstruction leads to a similar situation. Sonography is used for diagnosing oligohydramnios because of possible clinical complications. Amniotic fluid is swallowed by the fetus, about 400 ml/day near term. In esophageal atresia, the fetus is unable to swallow amniotic fluid, which accumulates because it cannot pass on to the stomach and intestines for absorption. An increase in the volume of amniotic fluid (>2000 ml) is poly-

hydramnios. Oligohydramnios may cause prematurity, fetal compression, and fetal anomalies, such as the amniotic band disruption complex (see Chapter 8). Meroanencephaly (anencephaly) and twin pregnancy are associated with polyhydramnios.

15. **B**   By 18 weeks, the fetus has a CRL of about 160 mm and its skin is covered with vernix caseosa; at 12 weeks the CRL is about 120 mm and at 22 weeks it is about 210 mm. At 18 weeks the fetus is not viable if born prematurely because its respiratory system is immature for gas exchanges. The presence of fingernails and toenails and open eyes are characteristics of a fetus that is at least 24 weeks old and viable.

16. **B**   Lanugo (downy hair) is usually absent in an infant with the postmaturity syndrome. These infants are thin and have a dry parchment skin but are often overweight. At birth, vernix caseosa is decreased or absent, and lanugo hair is lacking. The fingernails are long, and the infants show signs of increased alertness. Prolongation of pregnancy for 3 or more weeks beyond the expected date of confinement occurs in 5 to 6% of women. Some infants in prolonged pregnancies develop the postmaturity syndrome.

# *Five-Choice Association Questions*

**Directions:** Each group of questions below consists of a numbered list of descriptive words or phrases accompanied by a diagram with certain parts indicated by letters or by a list of lettered headings. For each numbered word or phrase, **select the lettered part or heading** that matches it correctly and then insert the letter in the space to the right of the appropriate number. Sometimes more than one numbered word or phrase may be correctly matched to the same lettered part or heading.

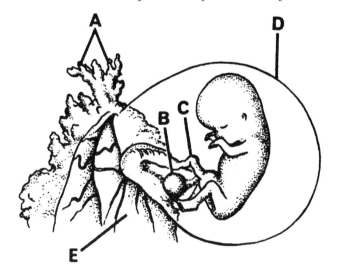

1. _____ Amniotic sac
2. _____ Contains umbilical vessels
3. _____ Chorionic sac
4. _____ Vestigial structure
5. _____ Chorionic villi
6. _____ Ensheathed by amnion

7. _____ Skin wrinkled and pink to red
8. _____ Quickening usually occurs
9. _____ Skeleton first shows clearly on radiographs and sonograms
10. _____ Sex is first distinguishable externally
11. _____ Eyebrows, head hair, and lanugo first visible
12. _____ Head constitutes about half of the fetus
13. _____ Fetus has good chance of surviving if born prematurely
14. _____ Brown fat begins to form
15. _____ Stage of initial activity of fetus

A. 12 weeks
B. 16 weeks
C. 20 weeks
D. 25 weeks
E. 29 weeks

## Answers and Explanations

1. **D**  The amniotic sac contains amniotic fluid, which permits free movement of the fetus and symmetric external growth. The fluid also cushions the fetus against jolts the mother may receive and helps to control the fetus's body temperature.

2. **C**  The umbilical cord contains umbilical vessels, normally two arteries and one vein. The vein carries nutrients and oxygenated blood to the fetus, and the arteries carry poorly oxygenated blood and waste products to the placenta, where the carbon dioxide and waste substances are transferred to the maternal blood for disposal.

3. **E**  The chorionic sac at this stage normally is embedded in the endometrium and contains the embryo in its amniotic sac. Chorionic villi cover most of the outer wall of the sac at this stage. Some villi have degenerated because they were compressed and received insufficient blood supply for survival.

4. **B**  The small remnant of the yolk sac indicated is a vestigial structure, serving no function at this stage. Part of the early yolk sac is incorporated into the embryo during the fourth week as the primordial gut. Within a few weeks, the remnant of the yolk sac indicated degenerates and disappears.

5. **A**  Chorionic villi project from the wall of the chorionic sac. These important parts of the placenta normally are embedded in the endometrium and bathed in maternal blood. It is through the villi that the exchange of nutrients between mother and fetus takes place.

6. **C**  The umbilical cord has an external investment of amnion. As the amniotic sac enlarges, the amnion gradually forms the outer covering of the cord.

7. **D**  During the 21- to 25-week period, the skin usually is wrinkled and pink to red because blood in the capillaries is visible through the thin, transparent skin. During the subsequent 4 weeks, considerable subcutaneous fat forms, smoothing out many of the wrinkles.

8. **C**  During the 17- to 20-week period, movements of the fetus — quickening — usually are felt by the mother for the first time. Although the fetus begins to move several weeks earlier, the movements are usually too slight to be felt by the mother.

9. **B**  Toward the end of the 13- to 16-week period, the skeleton clearly shows on radiographs (x-ray films). Care is taken to prevent the fetus from receiving too much radiation because of the possible adverse effects on its germ cells and developing brain. Sonography is widely used for examining the fetus.

10. **A**  Sex is first distinguishable during the 8- to 12-week period. At 8 weeks, the external genitalia of males and females appear similar. By the tenth week, it may be possible to differentiate between males and females, but the mature form of the genitalia is not reached until the 12th week.

11. **C**  The 17- to 20-week period is important for several reasons. Fetal movements are first felt by the mother; vernix caseosa forms and affords protection for the fetal skin; lanugo, head hair, and the eyebrows become visible, and brown fat begins to form. This specialized fat is an important site of heat production.

12. **A**  At the beginning of the fetal period, the head constitutes about half the length of the fetus. Thereafter, there is a relative slowdown in the growth of the head compared with the rest of the body. The large head in early fetuses results from the rapid development of the brain.

13. **E**  By the 26- to 29-week period, the fetus has a reasonably good chance of surviving if it is born prematurely, and is given intensive care; however, the mortality rate usually is high because of respiratory difficulties. The fetus is able to survive primarily because its respiratory and nervous systems have matured to the stage

where rhythmic breathing can occur. Capillary proliferation in the lungs becomes active during this period. Before the 26- to 28-week period, the pulmonary vascular bed is unable to accommodate the entire cardiac output and so gas exchange in the lungs may not be adequate to support life.

14. **C** Brown fat begins to form by the 20-week period. Heat is produced in this specialized adipose tissue, particularly during the newborn period, by oxidizing fatty acids. Brown fat is found chiefly at the root of the neck, posterior to the sternum, and in the perirenal regions.

15. **A** The stage of initial activity is during the 8- to 12-week period. By the end of 12 weeks, stroking the lips of a fetus causes it to begin sucking, and if the eyelids are stroked, there is a reflex response. These early movements of the fetus are too slight to be felt by the mother. She usually cannot detect fetal movements until the 17- to 20-week period; these movements — quickening — constitute a positive sign of a living fetus.

# Placenta and Fetal Membranes

## 7

## objectives

Be able to:

- Draw and label simple sketches showing the amnion, chorion, yolk sac, and allantois. Discuss the fate of yolk sac and allantois.
- Describe the development of the placenta, using drawings to show the essential features of placental structure and function.
- Illustrate the placental membrane, and discuss the transfer of materials between fetal and maternal blood streams.
- List the main activities of the placenta, discussing their role in maintaining pregnancy and promoting development.
- Draw and label simple sketches showing the gross and microscopic structure of the placenta and umbilical cord after birth.
- Illustrate with sketches and discuss the basis of multiple births.

## Five-Choice Completion Questions

**Directions:** Each of the following statements or questions is followed by five suggested responses or completions. **Select the one best answer** in each case.

1. Primary chorionic villi are first recognizable by the end of the _____ week.
   - A. first
   - B. second
   - C. third
   - D. fourth
   - E. fifth

2. The most distinctive characteristic of a primary chorionic villus is its
   - A. outer syncytial layer
   - B. cytotrophoblastic shell
   - C. mesenchymal core
   - D. core of cytotrophoblast
   - E. villous appearance

3. Villi are designated as secondary chorionic villi when they
   - A. contact the decidua basalis
   - B. are covered by syncytiotrophoblast
   - C. develop a mesenchymal core
   - D. have branch villi
   - E. develop capillaries

4. When chorionic villi are vascularized, they are called _____ villi.
   - A. branch
   - B. stem
   - C. tertiary
   - D. anchoring
   - E. true

5. The most important region of the placenta for nutrition of the embryo is the decidua _____.
   - A. vera
   - B. capsularis
   - C. parietalis
   - D. basalis
   - E. none of the above

6. Which of the following regions of the decidua degenerates and disappears during the second trimester of pregnancy?
   - A. decidua vera
   - B. decidua capsularis
   - C. decidua parietalis
   - D. decidua basalis
   - E. none of the above

7. Which of the following substances is least likely to be present in the intervillous space?
   - A. oxygen
   - B. carbon dioxide
   - C. maternal blood
   - D. fetal blood
   - E. electrolytes

8. Which of the following materials usually do not cross the placental membrane?
   - A. free fatty acids
   - B. steroid hormones
   - C. bacteria
   - D. vitamins
   - E. drugs

9. The substance exchanged most rapidly and freely between the mother and her embryo is
   - A. water
   - B. vitamins
   - C. antibodies
   - D. free fatty acids
   - E. minerals

10. The most characteristic feature of the maternal surface of the placenta is its
    - A. attachment of the cord
    - B. amniotic covering
    - C. cotyledons
    - D. shreds of decidua
    - E. intervillous spaces

11. At which of the following stages of development is division of embryonic material *not likely* to result in normal monozygotic twinning?
    - A. two-cell stage
    - B. morula
    - C. blastocyst
    - D. primitive streak
    - E. bilaminar embryo

12. An examination of the placenta and fetal membranes of male twins revealed two amnions, two chorions, and fused placentas. Twinning probably resulted from
    - A. dispermy
    - B. fertilization of two oocytes
    - C. superfecundation
    - D. fertilization of one oocyte
    - E. the effect of gonadotropins

13. With respect to dizygotic twins, which of the following is correct?
    - A. Result from the fertilization of two oocytes by two sperms
    - B. Result from the division of the embryoblast into two primordia
    - C. Usually begin to develop during the blastocyst stage
    - D. Usually are similar.
    - E. One chorionic sac is present.

14. Oligohydramnios was diagnosed in a near-term pregnant woman. What type of developmental defect might be present in the fetus?
    A. meroanencephaly
    B. renal agenesis
    C. esophageal atresia
    D. hyaline membrane disease
    E. absence of an umbilical artery

15. Fetal infection may result from the placental transfer of which of the following infectious agents?
    A. cytomegalovirus
    B. Rubella virus
    C. *Toxoplasma gondii*
    D. *Treponema pallidum*
    E. all of the above

16. Most drugs administered during pregnancy pass through the placental membrane by
    A. simple diffusion
    B. facilitated diffusion
    C. active transport
    D. pinocytosis
    E. none of the above

17. Which of the following *does not cross* the placental membrane?
    A. carbon monoxide
    B. thyroxine
    C. antibodies
    D. uric acid
    E. heparin

18. The average length of the umbilical cord at full term is _____ cm.
    A. 30–40
    B. 40–50
    C. 50–60
    D. 60–70
    E. 70–80

## Answers and Explanations

1. **B** The appearance of primary chorionic villi is a distinctive feature at the end of the second week. Commencing on about day 9 and continuing until the fourth week, there is intense growth and differentiation of the chorion.

2. **D** Early in the second week, irregular processes of syncytiotrophoblast form; outgrowths of cytotrophoblast soon extend into these processes. When these primordial villi acquire cores of cytotrophoblast, they are called primary chorionic villi. They represent the first stage in the development of the histological structure of the chorionic villi.

3. **C** The distinctive histological characteristic of a secondary chorionic villus is its core of mesenchyme. This embryonic connective tissue is derived from the extraembryonic somatic mesoderm. This change occurs at the end of the second week or early in the third week.

4. **C** The final stage in the elaboration of the histological structure of chorionic villi results in the formation of tertiary villi. These villi form the stem villi of the mature placenta. Sometimes the adjective true is used to describe villi in the final stage of development, but tertiary is the better term. The arteriocapillary venous system within the core of each villus develops by the end of the third week, and these vessels join those in the chorion, connecting stalk, and embryo. By the end of the third week, a simple placental circulation is established.

5. **D** The gravid endometrium underlying the conceptus — the decidua basalis — constitutes the maternal part of the placenta. The placenta is primarily an organ for the interchange of material between the maternal and fetal blood streams (e.g., oxygen, carbon dioxide, and food materials).

6. **B**  As the conceptus enlarges, the decidua capsularis bulges into the uterine cavity and becomes greatly attenuated. It eventually fuses with the decidua parietalis, obliterating the uterine cavity. By 22 weeks, reduced blood supply to the decidua capsularis results in its degeneration and subsequent disappearance.

7. **D**  There normally is no intermingling of fetal and maternal blood in the intervillous space. Small amounts of fetal blood may enter the maternal circulation through minute defects in the placental membrane. The circulation of maternal blood in the intervillous space is of particular importance in the supply of oxygen, electrolytes, and nutrient substances to the fetus and for the removal of waste products (e.g., carbon dioxide and urea).

8. **C**  Bacteria are not transferred across the placenta. Other microorganisms (e.g., rubella virus, cytomegalovirus, and *Toxoplasma gondii*) cross the placenta and cause congenital anomalies. When present in the maternal blood, bacteria may form the origin of an infection that subsequently may enter the fetal circulation. Almost all substances are probably able to cross the placenta to some extent. It is the rate and the mechanism of crossing that differ. The old sievelike concept of the placental membrane has been replaced by a more complex view in which the placenta selectively controls the rates of transfer of a wide variety of materials.

9. **A**  Water is readily transferred between the mother and her embryo or fetus and in increasing amounts as pregnancy progresses. Each solute transferred to the embryo and used liberates water molecules. Also, the oxidation of glucose and other nutrients results in the production of water molecules.

10. **C**  The 15 to 30 cotyledons give the maternal surface of the placenta a characteristic cobblestone appearance. The cotyledons are separated by grooves formerly occupied by the placental septa. Although shreds of the decidua basalis are attached to the surface of the cotyledons, they are clearly identifiable only under the microscope. The attachment of the umbilical cord and the amniotic covering are features of the fetal surface of the placenta.

11. **D**  After the end of the second week and establishment of a primitive streak, it is unlikely that separate monozygotic twins can develop. If partitioning of the embryonic disc during the second week is incomplete, conjoined twins result. Studies of the chorion, amnion, and placentas of monozygotic twins indicate that most partitioning of embryonic formative material occurs during the blastocyst stage, between days 4 and 7. Separation of the embryoblast into two parts results in the formation of two embryonic discs, two primitive streaks, and separate embryos.

12. **B**  The presence of two chorionic sacs usually indicates dizygotic (dissimilar or fraternal) twinning. From two-thirds to three-fourths of all human twins are dizygotic. The placentas and membranes observed could be associated with monozygotic twinning because in 25 to 30%, monozygotic twinning results from separation of the first two or more blastomeres. This results in the formation of two amniotic sacs and two chorionic sacs and separate or fused placentas. Thus, it may be difficult to determine if twins with the kind of membranes described are monozygotic or dizygotic. If they are of opposite sex or have different blood types, they are dizygotic. Like-sex twins, as in this case, may be considered monozygotic when they have the same blood type and strongly resemble each other in such characteristics as hair and eye color, fingerprints, and the shape of the external ear.

13. **A**  Dizygotic twins result from the fertilization of two oocytes by two sperms. The twins are genetically different and may be of the same sex or different sexes. Monozygotic twins usually develop from the two embryonic primordia formed as a result of the division of the embryoblast during the blastocyst stage. Monozygotic twins are genetically identical and of the same sex. Dizygotic twins have two amnions and two chorions, but the placentas may be fused. Each monozygotic twin has its own amniotic sac, but they share a common chorionic sac and placenta.

14. **B**  Oligohydramnios — low volume of amniotic fluid — results in most cases from placental insufficiency, which results in reduced placental

blood flow. Renal agenesis is the fetal defect usually associated with oligohydramnios because of the lack of fetal urine production. Urine makes a major contribution to the volume of amniotic fluid. A common cause of oligohydramnios is preterm rupture of the amniochorionic membrane. Meroanencephaly and esophageal atresia are associated with polyhydramnios (high volumes of amniotic fluid).

15. **E** Cytomegalovirus, rubella virus, and the microorganisms that cause syphillis (*Treponema pallidum*) and toxoplasmosis (*Toxoplasma gondii*) all cross the placenta and may infect the fetus. In some cases, congenital anomalies or death may occur, depending on the infectious agent and the stage of pregnancy.

16. **A** Most drugs are transported across the placental membrane from the mother to the embryo or fetus by simple diffusion. The placental transfer of a drug depends on its molecular weight, degree of ionization, and lipid solubility. Some drugs can affect the development of the embryo, leading to major congenital anomalies. Because of the potential risk of damaging the embryo, physicians must weigh the risk against the benefits when prescribing drugs to pregnant women.

17. **E** Heparin, an anticoagulant, is not transferred across the placental membrane. Oxygen, carbon dioxide, and carbon monoxide cross the placental membrane by simple diffusion. Thyroxine is essential for the development of the embryo/fetus and freely crosses the placental membrane. The nitrogenous waste products urea and uric acid readily cross the placental membrane by simple diffusion and are eventually excreted by the mother.

18. **C** The average length of the umbilical cord at full term is about 55 cm. The cord normally contains two arteries and one vein which transport gases, nutrients, and metabolic waste products between the mother and fetus. Doppler ultrasonography is used for assessing blood flow in the umbilical cord. Fetal complications may follow when the cord is very long or too short. For example, an excessively long cord may prolapse and the blood vessels become compressed, which leads to death of the fetus. A long cord may also become tightly coiled around the neck of the fetus, resulting in strangulation of the fetus due to compression of the umbilical vein. During delivery, a very short cord may result in premature separation of the placenta from its attachment to the endometrium.

## *Five-Choice Association Questions*

**Directions:** Each group of questions below consists of a numbered list of descriptive words or phrases accompanied by a diagram with certain parts indicated by letters or by a list of lettered headings. For each numbered word or phrase, **select the lettered part or heading** that matches it correctly and then insert the letter in the space to the right of the appropriate number. Sometimes more than one numbered word or phrase may be correctly matched to the same lettered part or heading.

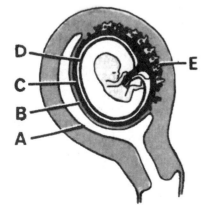

1. _____ Decidua capsularis
2. _____ Ensheaths umbilical cord
3. _____ Smooth chorion
4. _____ Decidua parietalis
5. _____ Fuses with decidua parietalis
6. _____ Maternal part of placenta

A. Separate placentas and membranes
B. Fibrinoid material
C. Amniochorionic membrane

D. Monochorionic placenta
E. Syncytial knot

7. _____ Occurs only in monozygotic twins
8. _____ Nuclear aggregation
9. _____ Unusual in monozygotic twins

10. _____ Stains intensely with eosin
11. _____ Extends into cervical canal during labor
12. _____ Forms on the surfaces of chorionic villi

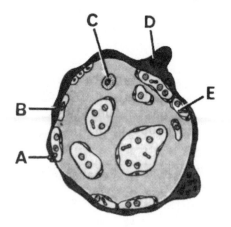

13. _____ Fetal capillary
14. _____ Macrophage
15. _____ Placental membrane
16. _____ Fetal blood
17. _____ Syncytial knot
18. _____ Fibrinoid material

A. Anchoring villi
B. Cytotrophoblast
C. Amnion
D. Battledore placenta
E. Cotyledons

19. _____ Fetal surface of placenta
20. _____ Largely disappears by birth
21. _____ Features of maternal surface of placenta
22. _____ Marginal attachment of umbilical cord
23. _____ Forms part of early placental membrane
24. _____ Places of attachment to decidua basalis

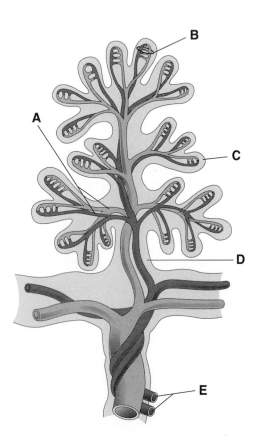

25. _____ Branch villus
26. _____ Fetal capillaries
27. _____ Syncytiotrophoblast
28. _____ Umbilical arteries
29. _____ Arteriocapillary venous network

## Answers and Explanations

1. **B** The decidua capsularis is the part of the decidua (gravid endometrium) that encapsulates the luminal surface of the implanted conceptus. At the stage shown, it is fused with the smooth chorion (chorion laeve). Together the amnion and chorion form the amniochorionic membrane.

2. **D** As the amniotic sac enlarges, it obliterates the chorionic cavity and ensheaths the umbilical cord. The amnion becomes the epithelial covering of the cord.

3. **C** The smooth chorion is continuous with the chorionic plate ("roof") of placenta. From the third to eighth week, the chorionic sac is covered by villi. The villi degenerate as the amniotic sac enlarges and presses the chorion against the decidua capsularis. This reduces the blood supply to the villi and results in their degeneration.

4. **A** The decidua parietalis refers to the endometrium lining parts of the uterus not directly involved with the conceptus (i.e., endometrium not designated as decidua capsularis or decidua basalis).

5. **B** The decidua capsularis enlarges with the growing conceptus and bulges into the uterine cavity. The decidua capsularis eventually fuses with the decidua parietalis, thereby obliterating the uterine cavity. By about 22 weeks, reduced blood supply to the attenuated decidua capsularis causes it to degenerate and gradually disappear.

6. **E** The decidua basalis forms the maternal part of the placenta. The fetal part is formed by the villous chorion (chorion frondosum). Together they form a unique fetomaternal organ, the placenta, the basic function of which is to bring the maternal and fetal circulations into proximity to permit effective exchange of materials.

7. **D** A monochorionic twin placenta, associated with twins in separate amniotic sacs, occurs only with monozygotic twins; thus, this type of placenta is diagnostic of monozygotic twinning. The twins often have a common fetal-placental circulation.

8. **E** At some sites, the syncytiotrophoblast of the placental membrane in mature placentas shows protuberances or sprouts of cytoplasm that contain aggregations of syncytiotrophoblastic nuclei — syncytial knots. Some knots break off and float in the intervillous space. They may pass into the maternal circulation through the uterine veins and lodge in the capillaries of the lungs. This occurrence is not usually considered to be of clinical significance because these nuclear masses are believed to degenerate and disappear.

9. **A** Monozygotic twins that develop after separation of the early blastomeres have separate placentas and membranes. Because the early blastocysts are enclosed in the same zona pellucida, they usually implant close together and their chorionic sacs and placentas usually fuse. This arrangement of the placentas and membranes commonly occurs with dizygotic twins. Thus, other criteria must be used to determine what type of twinning occurred (e.g., comparison of genetic markers such as blood groups or serum factors). A difference in any genetic marker indicates dizygosity. Similarities in several genetic markers do not prove monozygosity because any two children of the same parents might resemble each other in these genetic markers by chance. Many other genetic markers must then be studied before monozygosity is proved or highly probable.

10. **B** Fibrinoid material stains intensely with eosin in hematoxylin–eosin–stained sections of chorionic villi. It has been shown to be a mucoprotein–mucopolysaccharide complex. It is present in younger placentas but becomes increasingly abundant in older placentas. It appears at the junction between fetal and maternal tissues in the chorionic plate ("roof" of placenta), and on the surfaces of villi. Fibrinoid material is believed to be important in the prevention of rejection of the placenta and fetus by the mother. These age changes in

the material are closely linked with the functional efficiency of the placenta because this amorphous material reduces the surface area of the placental membrane available for exchange of materials.

11. **C** The chorion, with which the amnion is fused, extends into the cervical canal during the first stage of labor and helps to dilate the cervix. When the fused layers of amnion and chorion (amniochorionic membrane) rupture, the amniotic fluid escapes through the cervix and vagina.

12. **B** Fibrinoid is an eosinophilic, homogeneous substance that forms on the surfaces of chorionic villi and reduces the area of tissues through which exchange of materials between the maternal and fetal circulations may take place. It consists of fibrin and other unidentified substances.

13. **E** The fetal capillaries, embedded in the connective tissue of the chorionic villi, are part of an arteriocapillary–venous system that carries the fetal blood. As pregnancy advances, the capillaries increase in size and their walls eventually come into intimate relation with the syncytiotrophoblast. The endothelium of the capillary is separated from the syncytiotrophoblast by only an extremely delicate network of reticular fibers.

14. **C** The large cells in the mesenchymal core of chorionic villi are called Hofbauer cells. The vacuoles in these cells contain mucopolysaccharides, mucoproteins, and lipids. Although the complete role of these cells is not understood, they are thought to be macrophages.

15. **A** The placental membrane may be defined as the fetal tissues that are interposed between the fetal and placental circulations. The structure and thickness of the membrane vary at different stages of pregnancy. The placental membrane becomes extremely thin as pregnancy advances, and its permeability increases. The thickness of the membrane is also affected by the extent of distention of the capillaries in the villus.

16. **E** Poorly oxygenated blood passes from the fetus in the umbilical arteries. These arteries divide into a number of radially disposed vessels as the cord attaches to the placenta. The arterial branches pass into the chorionic villi and form an extensive arteriocapillary–venous system.

17. **D** Syncytial knots consist of aggregations of nuclei in protuberances of cytoplasm of the syncytiotrophoblast. They form at intervals along a villus; occasionally they break off and enter the maternal circulation. Apparently these nuclear aggregations have a short life in the maternal blood.

18. **B** Fibrinoid material develops as a homogeneous layer at various places on the maternal aspect of the villi. Because it is at the fetomaternal junction of tissues, fibrinoid is believed to be important in preventing rejection of the fetus by the mother. Composed of fibrin and other unidentified substances, fibrinoid decreases the permeability of the placental membrane for exchange of material between the fetal and maternal blood streams.

19. **C** The amnion adheres to the smooth fetal surface of the placenta and is continuous with the epithelial membrane covering the umbilical cord. The umbilical vessels radiate over the fetal surface of the placenta deep to the amnion.

20. **B** The cytotrophoblastic layer begins to retrogress and disappear at about 20 weeks. Some cells of this layer, however, persist until full term.

21. **E** Cotyledons are characteristic features of the maternal surface of the placenta. The placental septa divide the maternal surface into 15 to 30 cotyledons, which gives the expelled placenta a cobblestone appearance. During examination of the placenta after delivery, special attention should be given to determining whether the cotyledons are all present and intact. If they are not all recognizable and complete, placental tissue may still be in the uterus and must be removed.

22. **D** When the umbilical cord and vessels are attached to the margin of the placenta, it is called a battledore placenta because of its resemblance to the bat used in the medieval game of battledore and shuttlecock. This is a common variation of placental form. Battledore placenta (marginal insertion of cord) has some clinical significance because slight bleeding occasionally occurs. It has also been shown that many patients with battledore placentas have premature labor.

23. **B** The cytotrophoblast consists of large, pale cells with relatively large nuclei. Their cytoplasm contains vacuoles and some glycogen. The placenta synthesizes glycogen early in pregnancy, and its declining ability to perform this activity later in pregnancy may be related to the assumption of this function by the fetal liver and to the retrogression of the cytotrophoblast.

24. **A** The main means of attachment of the conceptus to the uterus is by anchoring stem villi that pass from the chorionic plate to the decidua basalis. Columns of cytotrophoblastic cells extend through the syncytiotrophoblast at the tips of these villi and cover the maternal tissue. Soon cytotrophoblastic cells from adjacent villi join to form a cytotrophoblastic shell around the conceptus. This shell is also attached to the decidua basalis.

25. **C** The main stem villi give rise to numerous branch villi that are bathed by maternal blood in the intervillous spaces. Exchange of gases, nutrients, and waste products between mother and fetus occurs between maternal blood in the intervillous space and fetal vessels in the branch villi.

26. **A** Fetal capillaries are tiny blood vessels in the branch villi that transport poorly oxygenated blood and waste products from the fetus and carry well oxygenated blood and nutrients to the fetus. Exchange of material occurs between the blood in the fetal capillaries and in the intervillous space.

27. **D** Cells from the cytotrophoblast proliferate rapidly, migrate into the syncytiotrophoblast, and lose their cell membrane. During implantation, the highly invasive syncytiotrophoblast invades the endometrial connective tissue and by the end of the second week the blastocyst is fully implanted in the endometrium.

28. **E** There are normally two umbilical arteries and one umbilical vein in the umbilical cord. The presence of only one umbilical artery may be associated with congenital anomalies in the fetus, often involving the heart and blood vessels. The umbilical arteries transport poorly oxygenated blood and waste products from the fetus to the placenta.

29. **B** An extensive arteriocapillary venous network is formed in the numerous villi from branches of the umbilical arteries and veins. Only the thin placental membrane separates fetal blood in the arteriocapillary venous plexus from the maternal blood in the intervillous space.

# Human Birth Defects

**8**

## Objectives

Be able to:

- Discuss birth defects with special reference to critical periods of development.
- Define the terms teratology and teratogens.
- Discuss the causes of congenital anomalies under each of the following headings, giving examples of their characteristic anomalous patterns:

  *Genetic Factors:* Changes in chromosome number (aneuploidy and polyploidy), structural abnormalities (translocation and deletion), and gene mutation

  *Environmental Factors:* Irradiation, infections, and drugs

  *Genetic and Environmental Factors:* Multifactorial inheritance

## Five-Choice Completion Questions

**Directions:** Each of the following statements or questions is followed by five suggested responses or completions. **Select the one best answer** in each case.

1. Major congenital anomalies are recognized in about _____% of neonates (newborns).
   - A. 0.5
   - B. 3.0
   - C. 6.0
   - D. 10
   - E. 15

2. What percentage of deaths in the neonatal period is attributed to major birth defects?
   - A. 2
   - B. 5
   - C. 15
   - D. 20
   - E. 25

3. Most major congenital anomalies result from
   - A. numerical chromosomal abnormalities
   - B. structural chromosomal abnormalities
   - C. mutant genes
   - D. infectious agents
   - E. unknown causes

4. The infectious agent most likely to cause a triad of congenital anomalies consisting of heart defects, cataracts, and deafness is
   - A. *Toxoplasma gondii*
   - B. varicella (chickenpox)
   - C. herpes zoster virus
   - D. rubella virus
   - E. cytomegalovirus

5. Which of the following microorganisms is unlikely to cause major congenital anomalies?
   A. *Treponema pallidum*
   B. cytomegalovirus
   C. varicella
   D. *Toxoplasma gondii*
   E. rubella virus

6. The frequency, severity, and type of defects produced by the rubella virus usually depend on the
   A. number of previous infections
   B. mother's age
   C. severity of the infection
   D. time of maternal infection
   E. sex and age of the embryo

7. Sex chromatin studies indicate that the frequency of sex chromatin – positive males in the general population is about 1:500. Chromosomal studies reveal that the most common chromosome complement (karyotype) in these males is
   A. 48, XXXY
   B. 47, XXY
   C. 48, XXYY
   D. 49, XXXYY
   E. 49, XXXXY

8. Late maternal age and nondisjunction of chromosomes during gametogenesis often are related. In which of the following syndromes is late maternal age believed to be a major factor?
   A. cri du chat syndrome
   B. Turner syndrome
   C. Klinefelter syndrome
   D. Edward syndrome
   E. Down syndrome

9. Congenital anomalies that result from chromosomal breakage are likely to occur in infants born to mothers who received or used
   A. lysergic acid (LSD)
   B. marijuana
   C. heroin
   D. radiation
   E. nonprescription drugs

10. Certain chemical agents exhibit varying degrees of teratogenicity when administered during the embryonic period. Which of the following substances is most likely to cause birth defects in human embryos?
    A. cortisone
    B. aminopterin
    C. potassium iodide
    D. lysergic acid
    E. aspirin

11. Infants with microcephaly are grossly retarded because brain development is rudimentary. The cause of this condition often is uncertain. From the list of known human teratogens, the most unlikely cause of microcephaly is
    A. rubella virus
    B. cytomegalovirus
    C. *Toxoplasma gondii*
    D. therapeutic radiation
    E. thalidomide

12. Environmental causes of human congenital anomalies may be prevented, to some extent, with proper counseling. An inappropriate medical advice to give a woman who has just missed a menstrual period and may be pregnant is to
    A. take only those drugs that have been prescribed by your doctor.
    B. avoid exposure to ionizing radiation.
    C. obtain a vaccination for protection against rubella infection.
    D. avoid people who have infectious diseases.
    E. eat a good-quality diet and do not smoke.

13. Growth deficiency, microcephaly, mental retardation, deafness, and chorioretinitis were observed in an infant during routine examination. Radiologic examination of the cranium revealed signs of cerebral calcification. The child's mother said that she had a viral infection during late pregnancy. Which of the following infectious agents is involved?

    A. herpes simplex virus
    B. varicella virus
    C. cytomegalovirus
    D. human immunodeficiency virus
    E. rubella virus

14. Which of the following drugs is unlikely to cross the placental membrane?

    A. heparin
    B. phenytoin
    C. retinoic acid
    D. insulin
    E. tetracycline

15. A 37-year-old woman gave birth to an infant with mental retardation and other anomalies, which included growth deficiency, microcephaly, short palpebral fissures, maxillary hypoplasia, and a thin upper lip. During her pregnancy, she drank both alcoholic beverages and coffee regularly and smoked more than a pack of cigarettes daily. Which of the following is probably responsible for the child's condition?

    A. mother's age
    B. alcohol ingestion
    C. cigarette smoking
    D. coffee
    E. genetic factors

16. Infants of mothers who smoke cigarettes heavily during pregnancy are most likely to have

    A. limb anomalies
    B. low birth weight
    C. ambiguous external genitalia
    D. facial anomalies
    E. spina bifida occulta

17. Which of the following teratogens is usually associated with tooth defects, such as discoloration of the teeth and hypoplasia of the enamel?

    A. cocaine
    B. alcohol
    C. thalidomide
    D. tetracyclines
    E. methotrexate

18. A pregnant woman ingested an androgenic substance throughout the first trimester. Exposure of the developing female fetus to excessive androgens may lead to

    A. labioscrotal fusion
    B. mental retardation
    C. intrauterine growth retardation
    D. cerebral calcification
    E. eye anomalies

19. A child with a congenital heart defect was born to a mother who took several drugs during pregnancy. As a causative factor of the infant's heart defect the attending doctor ruled out

    A. isotretinoin
    B. alcohol
    C. tetracyclines
    D. valproic acid
    E. lithium

20. Which of the following drugs/chemicals is (are) recognized as human teratogens?

    A. warfarin
    B. retinoic acid
    C. phenytoin
    D. tetracycline
    E. all of the above

## Answers and Explanations

1. **B** It is generally accepted that 3.0% neonates have a medically significant congenital defect. If one includes minor abnormalities, the incidence is about 5%. Not all defects are recognized at birth; indeed, if one includes all medically significant anomalies that are recognized by the end of the first year, the incidence increases to more than 6%. This emphasizes that less than half of all major birth defects are detected at birth.

2. **D** About 20% of deaths in the neonatal period can be attributed to the presence of birth defects (e.g., cardiac anomalies and defects of the central nervous system). More deaths occur in the first month of life than in the remaining months of the first year. Many abnormal fetuses can survive before birth but are unable to adjust to the profound changes associated with the onset of extrauterine life. Failure of the normal changes to occur in the circulatory system results in two of the most common congenital abnormalities of the heart and great vessels (patent oval foramen and patent ductus arteriosus). In many cases, these abnormalities can be corrected by surgical techniques.

3. **E** Most congenital anomalies result from unknown causes. Probably most birth defects are caused by an interaction of genetic and environmental factors (multifactorial inheritance). About 25% of anomalies are caused by genetic factors (A, B, and C), and the remaining anomalies are caused by environmental agents, such as the rubella virus and drugs.

4. **D** Rubella virus is a potent teratogen if present during early pregnancy. About 20% of mothers infected with rubella virus during the first month of pregnancy give birth to infants with birth defects. This is understandable because the heart, eyes, and internal ears are developing at this time. The risk of anomalies from infections during the second and third trimesters is low, but functional defects of the nervous system (e.g., mental retardation) and the internal ears may result from infections as late as the 25th week.

5. **C** Varicella virus may cross the placenta and infect the fetus; however, the defects are usually not severe. No maternal antibodies confer immunity on the fetus as occurs for smallpox. The other microorganisms listed all produce major congenital defects. Rubella virus produces its effects mainly during the embryonic period, whereas the syphilis organism, cytomegalovirus, and the parasite *Toxoplasma gondii* all produce their effects during the fetal period.

6. **D** The timing of a rubella infection during pregnancy is the most important factor. Infections early in pregnancy cause the most serious birth defects. Severe infections of the mother early in pregnancy often result in spontaneous abortion; milder infections may result in congenital anomalies.

7. **B** Newborn males with this sex chromosomal abnormality appear normal. During puberty, they develop the Klinefelter syndrome: small testes and hyalinization of the seminiferous tubules. Secondary sexual characteristics usually are poorly developed, and many of these males are tall and eunuchoid. Subnormal mentality is common, especially in people with more than three sex chromosomes. The chromosomal error (nondisjunction) that results in the Klinefelter syndrome typically occurs during the first meiotic division of maternal oogenesis, but it can occur during paternal spermatogenesis. In males with four X chromosomes, nondisjunction occurs during the first and second meiotic divisions.

8. **E** It is well established that the frequency of Down syndrome (trisomy 21) increases with maternal age. The frequency of this trisomy in mothers may be related to the circumstance that the primary oocytes are formed long before birth and remain in the first meiotic prophase until just before ovulation. There is no major maternal-age effect in the other syndromes listed.

9. **D** Most structural abnormalities result from chromosomal breaks induced by various en-

vironmental agents, especially high levels of ionizing radiation. Certain viruses have also been shown to cause fragmentation of chromosomes; however, there is no conclusive evidence that these chromosomal aberrations produce congenital defects. Similarly, it is known that LSD and marijuana may cause chromosomal damage, but there is no conclusive evidence to indicate that these drugs are teratogenic. Heroin is not known to cause chromosomal breakage, but it often causes narcotic addiction in neonates.

10. **B**  Aminopterin is a potent teratogen, as are other tumor-inhibiting chemicals (e.g., methotrexate). Potassium iodide may cause congenital goiter and the other substances listed may be weak teratogens, but there is not enough evidence to warrant inclusion of them in a list of known human teratogens.

11. **E**  Thalidomide is a highly potent teratogen, producing limb defects, deafness, and anomalies of the cardiovascular and digestive systems; however, it does not produce microcephaly, mental retardation, or other defects of the central nervous system. All the other environmental agents listed are known to cause microcephaly.

12. **C**  It would be inappropriate advice to recommend vaccination for any disease during early pregnancy. Although there is no conclusive information about the teratogenic potential of live attenuated rubella virus, it is contraindicated. Women should be immunized with live attenuated virus only when pregnancy is not planned during the next 2 months.

13. **C**  These are characteristic features of cytomegalovirus infection, which is the most common viral infection of the human fetus. Other findings may include blindness and hepatosplenomegaly, as well as audiologic and neurobehavioral disturbances.

14. **A**  Heparin is unlikely to cross the placental membrane. It is the drug of choice for pregnant women who require anticoagulant therapy. Molecular weight, degree of ionization, and lipid solubility are some factors that determine the placental transfer of a drug or chemical. The consumption of drugs during pregnancy is surprisingly high, and almost all drugs taken by the mother reach the embryo or fetus. Although relatively few drugs are proven human teratogens, possible adverse effects on the unborn child should be taken into consideration when drugs are used during pregnancy.

15. **B**  The findings in the infant are characteristic features of the fetal alcohol syndrome, now considered to be the most common cause of mental retardation in infancy. Although cigarette smoking is known to cause intrauterine growth retardation; however, like caffeine, there is no evidence that it is teratogenic in humans. Genetic factors are unlikely to be involved, and this case may require follow-up studies for appropriate counseling.

16. **B**  Maternal cigarette smoking is a well-established cause of intrauterine growth retardation (IUGR). Mothers who smoke 20 or more cigarettes daily may deliver prematurely, and their infants usually weigh less than normal. Maternal smoking is also associated with behavioral disturbances and decreased physical growth during childhood. Infants of mothers who stop smoking, especially before 16 weeks of gestation, show an improvement in their birth weights. There is little evidence in support of a strong association between maternal smoking and congenital anomalies. Nicotine, a vasoconstrictor, constricts the uterine blood vessels and reduces the transfer of oxygen and nutrients from the mother to the fetus. This leads to chronic hypoxia and IUGR.

17. **D**  Maternal use of tetracyclines during the second and third trimesters may cause a yellow to brown discoloration of the teeth and hypoplasia of the enamel of her fetus. Tetracyclines readily cross the placental membrane and are deposited in the bones and teeth of the fetus, with the potential to affect their growth. Because calcification of most permanent teeth begins at birth and is complete at about 8 years of age, tetracycline therapy during early childhood should be avoided. Maternal use of cocaine, thalidomide, alcohol, and methotrexate is not usually associated with tooth anomalies.

18. **A**  Fetuses who are normal 46, XX females may appear masculinized at birth because of

in utero exposure to androgens and high doses of progestogens during the first trimester of pregnancy. There is a varying degree of labio-scrotal fusion, and enlargement of the clitoris. Mental retardation, IUGR, and eye anomalies are associated with several teratogens, such as alcohol and the rubella virus. Cerebral calcification is usually present in an infant infected in utero with the intracellular parasite *Toxoplasma gondii* or with cytomegalovirus.

19. **C**  Congenital anomalies of the heart are more often found in infants exposed in utero to isotretinoin, alcohol, valproic acid, and lithium. Tetracyclines cause discoloration of teeth but are not known to cause heart defects.

20. **E**  All the substances listed are well documented as teratogens in humans. Their use during pregnancy is contraindicated, and inappropriate administration of these drugs could have legal consequences involving the physician. Usually the benefits of a particular drug are weighed against possible risks. Warfarin causes nasal hypoplasia, stippled epiphyses, eye anomalies, and mental retardation in the newborn. Retinoic acid induces craniofacial anomalies, mental retardation, and cardiovascular anomalies. Phenytoin is associated with IUGR, mental retardation, cleft palate, and pharyngeal hypoplasia. Tetracycline, which affects the fetus, causes stained teeth and hypoplasia of enamel.

# Five-Choice Association Questions

**Directions:** Each group of questions below consists of a numbered list of descriptive words or phrases. For each numbered word or phrase, **select the lettered part or heading** that matches it correctly and then insert the letter in the space to the right of the appropriate number. Sometimes more than one numbered word or phrase may be correctly matched to the same letter.

A. 47, XXX  
B. 45, XO  
C. Trisomy 18  
D. Trisomy 21  
E. 47, XXY  

1. _____ Webbed neck and short stature
2. _____ Mental retardation, low-set ears, and early postnatal death
3. _____ Normal female appearance and usually fertile
4. _____ Small testes and hyalinization of the seminiferous tubules
5. _____ The most common numerical autosomal abnormality
6. _____ Female with chromatin – negative nuclei
7. _____ Strong association with late maternal age
8. _____ Mental retardation, simian crease, and heart defect
9. _____ Sterile male with chromatin – positive nuclei

A. Cytomegalovirus  
B. Androgenic agents  
C. Thalidomide  
D. *Toxoplasma gondii*  
E. Aminopterin  

10. _____ Antitumor agent and potent teratogen
11. _____ Intracellular parasite often found in cats
12. _____ Potent teratogen that affects limb development
13. _____ May cause masculinization of female fetuses

14. _____ Known to cause meroanencephaly
15. _____ Mother may be infected with it by eating poorly cooked meat

## *Answers and Explanations*

1. **B** Webbed neck and short stature are associated with Turner syndrome (ovarian dysgenesis). These females have 44 autosomes and only 1 X chromosome. In the newborn period, these infants usually exhibit marked edema of the feet and webbing of the neck. The ovaries commonly consist of only connective tissue streaks. This condition is not recognized in many of these girls until they reach puberty (12 to 15 years), at which time they seek medical advice about primary amenorrhea (failure of menstruation to begin) and the lack of secondary sex development.

2. **C** Infants with trisomy 18 have multiple major anomalies. Like those with the less common trisomy 13 syndrome, these infants have a severe mental defect and die during early infancy. Trisomy 18 is much more severe than Down syndrome, and an excess of females are affected (about 78%).

3. **A** Most females with the triple X chromosome abnormality appear normal and are fertile. These women have two sex chromatin masses in their cells because of the presence of the extra X chromosome. Some triple X females have borne children, all of whom are normal and have normal karyotypes. Most females with four or more X chromosomes are also physically normal but severely retarded.

4. **E** XXY males appear normal at birth. Small testes and hyalinization of the seminiferous tubules are the constant characteristics of postpubertal XXY males with Klinefelter syndrome. The secondary sexual characteristics usually are poorly developed, and many of these males are tall and eunuchoid. Subnormal mentality is common.

5. **D** Trisomy 21 is the most common type of numerical autosomal abnormality, occurring about once in 600 neonates. The cause of the chromosomal abnormality (trisomy of chromosome 21) is nondisjunction during oogenesis, usually in older mothers. About 4% of people with Down syndrome have the extra 21 chromosome attached to another chromosome (usually number 14).

6. **B** Females with Turner syndrome (45, XO) were among the first cases studied when accurate chromosomal analyses became possible in 1958. Sex chromatin studies had shown a few years earlier that these females had chromatin-negative nuclei. Some females with stigmata of Turner syndrome are chromatin positive because they are mosaics (i.e., they have a 45, X cell line and a normal 46, XX cell line).

7. **D** Infants with Down syndrome are usually born to older mothers. The mean maternal age is about 35 years compared with 28 in a control population. The older name for this condition is mongolism, coined because of the somewhat slanting look of the eyes. It is an inappropriate name and should not be used.

8. **D** Infants with Down syndrome are mentally retarded (I.Q. commonly is in the 25 to 50 range) and have heart defects. The single transverse crease (simian crease) in place of the usual curved crease is found in about 50% of people with the syndrome. It is also found in people with other chromosomal abnormalities and in about 1% of normal people. The presence of a simian crease does not necessarily indicate a chromosomal abnormality and Down syndrome, but it is a useful criterion when associated with other characteristics (mental retardation hypotonia, epicanthal folds, furrowed and protruding tongue).

9. **E** Males with chromatin – positive nuclei have Klinefelter syndrome or a related condition. Newborn males appear normal, but the testes remain abnormally small as puberty

approaches owing to hyalinization of the seminiferous tubules. Consequently, they are sterile. Secondary sexual characteristics develop poorly, and gynecomastia (enlargement of breasts) may occur. These men typically are tall and eunuchoid and may have a subnormal mentality.

10. **E** Aminopterin, an antitumor agent, is also a potent human teratogen. Methotrexate, a derivative of aminopterin, is also teratogenic. These agents produce a wide range of severe skeletal defects and anomalies of the central nervous system (CNS). Aminopterin may produce meroanencephaly (anencephaly), intrauterine growth retardation, and many other CNS abnormalities.

11. **D** *Toxoplasma gondii* is an intracellular parasite. It infects many birds and mammals (especially cats), in addition to some humans. Toxoplasmosis, the disease caused by this microorganism, can be contracted from eating raw meat or through contact with infected animals (e.g., rabbits). The parasite affects the fetus during the second and third trimesters, producing microcephaly, microphthalmia, hydrocephaly, and chorioretinitis.

12. **C** Thalidomide produces severe limb anomalies in the embryo if taken by the mother during the first trimester. As little as 200 mg of this sedative and antinauseant may cause limb defects, cardiac defects, and ear anomalies.

13. **B** Androgenic agents and certain progestins administered to prevent abortion may cause masculinization of female fetuses. The substances known to cause these anomalies are ethisterone and norethisterone. All substances with known androgenic properties may cause masculinization if administered during the early part of the first trimester of pregnancy.

14. **E** Aminopterin, an antitumor agent and teratogen, is known to cause meroanencephaly (partial absence of the brain) if administered during the early period of brain development (third to fourth week).

15. **D** A mother may become infected with the parasite *Toxoplasma gondii* by eating raw or poorly cooked meat (e.g., rabbit) that contains the microorganism. She may contract toxoplasmosis from infected birds, animals, or people. If the parasite crosses the placental membrane, it causes maldevelopment during the fetal period. It causes microcephaly, microphthalmia, hydrocephaly, and chorioretinitis. There is no proof that the parasite affects development during organogenesis (i.e., during the embryonic period).

# Body Cavities, Mesenteries, and Diaphragm

## 9

### Objectives

Be able to:

- Describe, with the aid of diagrams, the development of the intraembryonic coelom and the changes resulting in it from longitudinal and transverse folding of the embryo during the fourth week.
- Give an account of the subdivision of the body cavities into the pericardial cavity, the pleural cavities, and the peritoneal cavity.
- Explain, with the aid of diagrams, the formation of the dorsal and ventral mesenteries.
- Describe the development of the diaphragm. Discuss its four components, positional changes, and innervation.
- Explain the embryological basis of congenital diaphragmatic hernia. Discuss the effects of this defect on the initiation of respiration at birth.

## Five-Choice Completion Questions

**Directions:** Each of the following statements or questions is followed by five suggested responses or completions. **Select the one best answer** in each case.

1. Autopsy of a newborn infant revealed a defect in the central part of the diaphragm and the presence of intestine in the thoracic cavity. The central tendon of the diaphragm is derived from the
   A. lateral body wall
   B. pleuroperitoneal membranes
   C. septum transversum
   D. pleuropericardial membranes
   E. esophageal mesentery

2. The intraembryonic coelom (embryonic body cavity) is first recognizable during the _____ week after fertilization.
   A. second
   B. third
   C. fourth
   D. fifth
   E. sixth

3. The first component of the primordial diaphragm is present at the end of the _____ week of development.
   A. second
   B. third
   C. fourth
   D. fifth
   E. sixth

4. After folding of the embryo, the dorsal mesentery extends from the
   A. cranial part of the foregut to the caudal region
   B. cranial part of the esophagus to the cloacal region
   C. caudal part of the esophagus to the cloacal region
   D. caudal part of the foregut to the cranial part of the hindgut
   E. stomodeum to the proctodeum (anal pit)

5. Failure of closure of the cranial end of a pericardioperitoneal canal results in communication between the pleural cavity on the affected side and the
   A. peritoneal cavity
   B. pericardial cavity
   C. abdominopelvic cavity
   D. other pleural cavity
   E. pelvic cavity

6. Failure of closure of the caudal end of a pericardioperitoneal canal results in communication between the pleural cavity on the affected side and the
   A. peritoneal cavity
   B. pericardial cavity
   C. abdominopelvic cavity
   D. other pleural cavity
   E. pelvic cavity

7. In a 4-week embryo, the developing diaphragm is located at the level of the
   A. superior cervical somites
   B. inferior thoracic somites
   C. superior thoracic somites
   D. superior lumbar somites
   E. inferior lumbar somites

8. Most muscle-forming cells that give rise to the musculature of the diaphragm are derived from mesenchymal cells that originate in the
   A. septum transversum
   B. cervical somites
   C. thoracic somites
   D. lumbar somites
   E. lateral mesoderm

9. The septum transversum gives rise to _____ of the diaphragm.
   A. small intermediate parts
   B. the right and left crura
   C. the central tendon
   D. posterolateral parts
   E. peripheral parts

10. In the 5-week embryo, the ventral mesentery of the primordial gut persists where it is attached to the
    A. primordial pharynx
    B. embryonic part of yolk stalk
    C. caudal region of hindgut
    D. caudal region of foregut
    E. cranial region of midgut

11. A congenital diaphragmatic hernia was diagnosed prenatally by ultrasonography. Which of the following structures was probably involved?
    A. septum transversum
    B. costodiaphragmatic recess
    C. pleuroperitoneal membrane
    D. dorsal mesentery of esophagus
    E. lateral body wall

12. Surrounding the chorion is the
    A. peritoneal cavity
    D. left pericardioperitoneal canal
    B. extraembryonic coelom
    E. pericardial cavity
    C. right pericardioperitoneal canal

13. The intraembryonic coelom is connected with the extraembryonic coelom until the _____ week, after which they become separated.
    A. 6th
    B. 8th
    C. 10th
    D. 12th
    E. 14th

## Answers and Explanations

1. **C** The septum transversum is the primordium of the central tendon of the diaphragm. The pleuropericardial membranes are not involved in the formation of the diaphragm. They form partitions at the cranial ends of the pericardioperitoneal canals and separate the pericardial cavity from the pleural cavities. The septum transversum, lateral body wall, pleuroperitoneal membranes, and esophageal mesentery are the main components of the developing diaphragm.

2. **B** Intercellular spaces, lined by mesothelium, appear in the lateral mesoderm and cardiogenic mesoderm 18 to 19 days after fertilization. These spaces coalesce to form the intraembryonic coelom (embryonic body cavity), a horseshoe-shaped cavity within the lateral and cardiogenic mesoderm in the embryo.

3. **B** The septum transversum is the first recognizable component of the developing diaphragm. It appears at the end of the third week as a mass of mesoderm cranial to the pericardial coelom. After the head fold occurs during the fourth week, the septum transversum forms a thick mass of mesenchyme between the thoracic and abdominopelvic cavities. Later it is invaded by the developing liver and eventually becomes a thin layer (primordium of central tendon of diaphragm) between the pericardial cavity and the liver.

4. **C** The dorsal mesentery extends from the caudal part of the esophagus to the cloacal region of the hindgut. In the region of the esophagus, the mesentery is called the mesoesophagus; in the stomach region, it is called the dorsal mesogastrium or greater omentum; and in the region of the colon, it is called mesocolon. The dorsal mesentery of the jejunum and ileum is called the mesentery proper. The dorsal mesentery of the duodenum (dorsal mesoduodenum) disappears completely, except near the pylorus of the stomach.

5. **B** Defective formation and/or fusion of the pleuropericardial membrane, usually on the left side, is uncommon. When this occurs, there is a defect in the fibrous pericardium, the adult derivative of the pleuropericardial membranes. Part of the left atrium may herniate into the left pleural cavity when there is a defect in the pericardium.

6. **A** Defective formation and/or fusion of the pleuroperitoneal membrane, usually on the left side, is relatively common (about once in 2200 births). This defect results in a posterolateral defect in the diaphragm through which abdominal viscera may herniate into the thorax. Congenital diaphragmatic hernia usually constitutes a medical-surgical emergency in the newborn period because of respiratory disorders (pressure on lungs, causes poor lung expansion and difficult breathing).

7. **A** As the head fold forms, the septum transversum and pericardial cavity move into a

ventral position. When it lies opposite to the upper cervical segments of the spinal cord, nerves from the third, fourth, and fifth segments grow into the septum transversum, forming the phrenic nerves. These nerves are the sole motor nerve supply to the diaphragm and are sensory to the central part of the diaphragm. In the later weeks of development, the diaphragm descends, so that the dorsal part reaches the level of the first lumbar vertebra by the end of the embryonic period.

8. **B**   Most of the musculature of the diaphragm is derived from mesenchymal cells that originate in the myotome regions of the cervical somites. When these cells migrate into the septum transversum with the developing phrenic nerves, they differentiate into myoblasts (developing muscle fibers). When the developing diaphragm migrates caudally during subsequent development, the phrenic nerves supplying these muscles follow the diaphragm caudally. Some myoblasts later differentiate from mesenchymal cells in the septum transversum. Other myoblasts probably arise from mesenchymal cells that migrate from the thoracic somites and enter the diaphragm with the lateral body wall tissues that split off as the pleural cavities enlarge by invading the chest wall.

9. **C**   The septum transversum gives rise to the central tendon of the diaphragm. Small intermediate parts of it are derived from the pleuroperitoneal membranes, and the crura develop from the growth of muscle fibers into the dorsal mesentery of the esophagus. The peripheral portions of the diaphragm are derived from lateral body wall tissue that is split off as the lungs and pleural cavities enlarge and burrow into the lateral body walls.

10. **D**   The ventral mesentery disappears except where it is attached to the caudal part of the foregut. This region gives rise to the terminal part of the esophagus, the stomach, and the superior (first) part of the duodenum. Caudal to the bile duct, the intestines have no ventral mesentery. When most of the ventral mesentery disappears, the right and left peritoneal cavities become a continuous large peritoneal sac — the peritoneal cavity — in which the viscera are suspended by the dorsal mesentery.

11. **C**   Congenital diaphragmatic hernia (CDH) usually results from failure of a pleuroperitoneal membrane to fuse with the dorsal mesentery of the esophagus and the septum transversum. Posterolateral defect of the diaphragm is the most common anomaly of the diaphragm. It usually occurs on the left side. This defect permits herniation of abdominal viscera into the thoracic cavity, which causes compression and hypoplasia of the lung. The prognosis is poor because of the resulting severe respiratory distress and other complications.

12. **B**   The extraembryonic coelom is a large cavity formed within the extraembryonic mesoderm during the second week. It surrounds the yolk sac and chorion. The extraembryonic coelom is not derived from the intraembryonic coelom, even though they communicate with each other. The intraembryonic coelom arises during the third week from isolated coelomic spaces in the lateral mesoderm and in the cardiogenic mesoderm. These spaces coalesce to form a horseshoe-shaped cavity that gives rise to the large peritoneal cavity, the two pericardioperitoneal canals (future pleural cavities), and the pericardial cavity.

13. **C**   The peritoneal part of the intraembryonic coelom becomes separated from the extraembryonic coelom in the 10th week. The intraembryonic coelom gives rise to the peritoneal cavity, the pleural cavities, and the pericardial cavity. The distal end of each limb of the horseshoe-shaped intraembryonic coelom opens into the extraembryonic coelom at the lateral edges of the embryonic disc. This communication is important because the midgut normally herniates through it into the umbilical cord, where the midgut develops into most of the small and large intestine. During the 10th week, as the intestine returns to the abdomen from the umbilical cord, the peritoneal cavity is separated from the extraembryonic coelom.

# Five-Choice Association Questions

**Directions:** Each group of questions below consists of a numbered list of descriptive words or phrases accompanied by a diagram with certain parts indicated by letters or by a list of lettered headings. For each numbered word or phrase, **select the lettered part or heading** that matches it correctly and then insert the letter in the space to the right of the appropriate number. Sometimes more than one numbered word or phrase may be correctly matched to the same lettered part or heading.

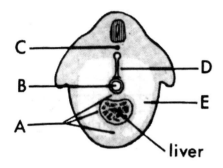

1. _____ Disappears caudally
2. _____ Derived from intraembryonic coelom
3. _____ Ventral mesentery of stomach
4. _____ Caudal part of foregut
5. _____ Dorsal mesogastrium

A. Costodiaphragmatic recess
B. Cervical myotomes
C. Congenital hiatal hernia
D. Pleuroperitoneal membrane
E. Pericardioperitoneal canal

6. _____ Large esophageal opening
7. _____ Extension of pleural cavity
8. _____ Posterolateral diaphragmatic defect
9. _____ Diaphragmatic muscles
10. _____ Connects the pericardial and peritoneal cavities
11. _____ Herniation of abdominal viscera

A. Esophageal mesentery
B. Pleuropericardial membrane
C. Phrenic nerves
D. Crura of diaphragm
E. Embryonic mediastinum

12. _____ Derived from third to fifth cervical spinal cord segments
13. _____ Common cardinal vein
14. _____ Muscular origins of diaphragm
15. _____ Mesenchyme separating lungs
16. _____ Forms median part of diaphragm

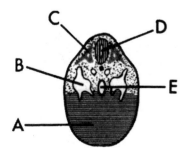

17. _____ Future pleural cavity
18. _____ Primordium of esophagus
19. _____ Produces mesenchyme
20. _____ Gives rise to central tendon
21. _____ Located caudal to heart

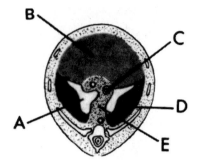

22. _____ Pleuroperitoneal membrane
23. _____ Derived from foregut
24. _____ Esophageal mesentery
25. _____ Future pleural cavity
26. _____ Gives rise to central tendon of
         diaphragm

## Answers and Explanations

1. **A**  The ventral mesentery disappears caudal to the superior or first part of the duodenum. Note that the liver is developing between the layers of the ventral mesentery. The ventral mesentery forms during transverse folding of the embryo and gives rise to the lesser omentum, falciform ligament, and visceral peritoneum of the liver.

2. **E**  The peritoneal cavity is derived from the caudal extension of the horseshoe-shaped intra-embryonic coelom that forms early in the fourth week of development. In the illustration, the foregut (primordial stomach) is suspended in the peritoneal cavity by the dorsal mesentery (dorsal mesogastrium) and the ventral mesentery (hepatogastric ligament).

3. **A**  The ventral mesentery of the stomach develops from the septum transversum and extends from this septum to the ventral aspect of the caudal part of the foregut. This part of the foregut gives rise to the stomach and the superior part of the duodenum. After the liver develops, the ventral mesentery attaches the stomach to the liver (hepatogastric ligament) and the first part of the duodenum to the liver (hepatoduodenal ligament).

4. **B**  The endoderm of the caudal part of the foregut gives rise to the epithelium and glands of the inferior end of the esophagus, the stomach, and the superior part of the duodenum. The muscular and fibrous elements of these structures are derived from the surrounding splanchnic mesoderm. The superior part of the foregut gives rise to the pharynx and its deriva-

tives, the lower respiratory tract, and the superior part of the esophagus.

5. **D**  The dorsal mesentery (dorsal mesogastrium) suspends the stomach in the peritoneal cavity. The spleen subsequently develops between the two layers of the dorsal mesogastrium. Later, as the result of positional changes and growth, the dorsal mesogastrium hangs over the transverse colon and small intestine; this part of the dorsal mesentery is the greater omentum.

6. **C**  If the embryonic esophageal hiatus or opening in the diaphragm is excessively large, abdominal viscera may herniate through it into the thorax, producing a congenital hiatal hernia (CDH). Another uncommon type of CDH, the hernia, is believed to be caused by a short esophagus. Because of this anomaly, the superior part of the stomach remains in the thorax and the stomach is constricted where it passes through the esophageal opening.

7. **A**  As the pleural cavities enlarge, they extend into the body walls, forming costodiaphragmatic recesses. This excavation process also splits off body wall tissue, which contributes to peripheral parts of the diaphragm and establishes the characteristic dome-shaped configuration of the diaphragm.

8. **D**  If the pleuroperitoneal membrane fails to develop or to fuse with other parts of the diaphragm, a posterolateral defect develops, usually on the left side. Associated with this defect is herniation of abdominal viscera into the thorax and compression of the lungs. This type of CDH

often results in a medical-surgical emergency because of difficulty in fetal breathing.

9. **B**  The diaphragmatic muscles are mainly derived from myoblasts that migrate from the myotome regions of the cervical somites. Other myoblasts are derived from the myotome regions of the thoracic somites, and some myoblasts originate in the body wall tissues.

10. **E**  The pericardioperitoneal canals become the adult pleural cavities. Membranes develop at the cranial and caudal ends of these canals that separate the pleural cavities from the pericardial cavity and the peritoneal cavity, respectively. The developing lungs invaginate the medial walls of the pericardioperitoneal cavities. The inner (visceral) and outer (parietal) walls of these canals eventually come close together as the layers of pleura.

11. **D**  Herniation of abdominal viscera into the thorax occurs through a posterolateral defect in the diaphragm where there is failure of development and/or fusion of the pleuroperitoneal membrane with other parts of the diaphragm, usually on the left side. Because of the presence of abdominal viscera in the thorax, the lungs often are compressed and may be hypoplastic (incompletely developed).

12. **C**  The phrenic nerves are derived from the third, fourth, and fifth cervical segments of the spinal cord. These nerves accompany the myoblasts that grow into the developing diaphragm from the myotome regions of the cervical somites. The diaphragm descends as elongation of the neck, descent of the heart, and expansion of the pericardial and pleural cavities occur. The descent of the diaphragm, after it receives its main nerve supply, explains the rather unusual course of the phrenic nerves.

13. **B**  The common cardinal veins — the main venous channels entering the heart — are in the pleuropericardial membranes. At first, these membranes appear as small ridges projecting into the pericardioperitoneal canals. They eventually fuse with the mesoderm ventral to the esophagus (primordial mediastinum), closing the connections between the pericardial cavity and the pleural cavities.

14. **D**  The crura of the diaphragm (muscular origins of diaphragm from superior lumbar vertebrae) develop as muscle fibers in the esophageal mesentery.

15. **E**  The mediastinum (median septum) in the embryo consists of a mass of embryonic connective tissue separating the lungs and extending from the sternum to the vertebral column. It forms the median dividing wall of the thoracic cavity and contains all the thoracic viscera and structures except the lungs.

16. **A**  The dorsal mesentery of the esophagus (mesoesophagus) forms the median part of the diaphragm. The pleuroperitoneal membranes fuse with the esophageal mesentery and septum transversum during the sixth week, forming a partition between the thoracic and abdominal cavities. Completion of the diaphragm occurs during the 9th to 12th weeks as body wall tissue is added to it peripherally.

17. **B**  The pericardioperitoneal canals are the future pleural cavities. As the lungs develop, they invaginate (push into) the medial walls of these canals, like fists pushed into the sides of almost empty balloons. These invaginations are so complete that the space between the two walls of the canals (future layers of pleura) is reduced to a narrow gap.

18. **E**  The foregut gives rise to the epithelium and glands of the esophagus and stomach. Other regions of the foregut give rise to the pharynx and its derivatives, lower respiratory tract, duodenum as far as the bile duct, liver, pancreas, and biliary apparatus.

19. **C**  The somites, derived by division of the paraxial mesoderm, give rise to the mesenchyme that differentiates into most of the axial skeleton and its associated musculature. Mesenchyme is an embryonic connective tissue that gives rise to a wide variety of adult tissues (e.g., fibroblasts, fibrocytes, osteoblasts, osteocytes, chondroblasts, chondrocytes, myoblasts, and muscle fibers).

20. **A**  The septum transversum, a thick mass of mesenchyme, gives rise to the central tendon of the diaphragm. It is the first component of

the diaphragm that is recognizable (end of third week). It forms the caudal limit of the pericardial cavity after folding of the embryo and separates it from the future peritoneal cavity. During the fourth week, groups of myoblasts (muscle-forming cells) from the cervical somites (three to five) migrate into the cranial part of the septum transversum, carrying their phrenic nerve fibers with them.

21. **A**  The septum transversum is located caudal to the heart. Early in the fourth week, it lies cranial to the pericardial coelom and primordial heart. As the brain develops, the head folds ventrally, carrying the septum transversum, developing heart, pericardial coelom, and the oropharyngeal membrane ventral to the foregut.

22. **D**  The pleuroperitoneal membranes, produced as the lungs and pleural cavities expand by invading the body walls, form caudal partitions in the pericardioperitoneal canals. These membranes gradually grow medially and fuse during the sixth week with the dorsal mesentery of the esophagus and the septum transversum to form the diaphragm. Failure of one of these membranes to form results in a CDH through which the abdominal viscera can herniate. The defect usually appears in the region of the left kidney.

23. **C**  The epithelium and glands of the esophagus are derived from the foregut. The muscular and fibrous elements are derived from the surrounding splanchnic mesenchyme. The foregut also gives rise to the epithelium and glands of the lower respiratory tract. Faulty partitioning of the foregut into the esophagus and trachea during the fourth and fifth weeks results in a tracheoesophageal fistula.

24. **E**  The esophageal mesentery (dorsal mesentery of esophagus) is one of the components of the primordial diaphragm. The other components are the septum transversum and pleuroperitoneal membranes. Later, a fourth component, the body wall, contributes to peripheral regions of the diaphragm. The esophageal mesentery constitutes the median portion of the diaphragm. The crura of the diaphragm develop from muscle fibers that form in the dorsal mesentery of the esophagus.

25. **A**  The pericardioperitoneal canals become the pleural cavities. The bronchial buds grow laterally during the fifth week and evaginate the medial walls of the canals. The inner walls of the canals become the visceral pleura and the outer walls become the parietal pleura.

26. **B**  The septum transversum gives rise to the central tendon of the diaphragm. Although initially located opposite the cervical region of the spinal cord, the septum transversum is invaded by myoblasts from the third, fourth, and fifth myotome regions of the cervical somites. Later, the diaphragm descends until its dorsal part lies at the level of the first lumbar vertebra. Thus, the seemingly curious origin and course of the phrenic nerves result from the developmental origin of the septum transversum.

# *Pharyngeal Apparatus*

**10**

## Objectives

Be able to:

- Explain what is meant by the term pharyngeal apparatus.
- List and illustrate the components of the pharyngeal arches.
- Construct and label diagrams showing the derivatives of the pharyngeal arch cartilages.
- Discuss the formation of the pharyngeal pouches, indicating their adult derivatives.
- Describe the development of the tongue and thyroid gland.
- Discuss the embryological basis of ectopic thyroid gland and thyroglossal duct cysts and sinuses.
- Illustrate the development of the face and palate, describing the embryological basis of cleft lip and cleft palate.
- Discuss the embryological basis of branchial cysts, sinuses, and fistulas; first arch syndrome; and DiGeorge syndrome.

## *Five-Choice Completion Questions*

**Directions:** Each of the following statements or questions is followed by five suggested responses or completions. **Select the one best answer** in each case.

1. The pharyngeal apparatus is composed of
   - A. pharyngeal grooves
   - B. pharyngeal arches
   - C. pharyngeal pouches
   - D. pharyngeal membranes
   - E. all of the above

2. The third pharyngeal arch cartilages give rise to which of the following structures?
   - A. stylohyoid ligament
   - B. thyroid cartilage
   - C. styloid process
   - D. sphenomandibular ligament
   - E. greater horns of hyoid bone

3. Which of the following structures *is not related* to the first pharyngeal arch?
   - A. malleus
   - B. facial nerve
   - C. Meckel cartilage
   - D. mandibular prominence
   - E. maxillary prominence

4. Which of the following structures *is not derived* from the second pharyngeal arch cartilage?
   - A. incus
   - B. stapes
   - C. styloid process
   - D. lesser horn of hyoid bone
   - E. superior part of hyoid bone

5. Pharyngeal arches are first recognizable around the middle of the _____ week of development.
   A. second
   B. third
   C. fourth
   D. fifth
   E. sixth

6. The cartilages of the larynx are derived mainly from the cartilages of which of the following pharyngeal arches?
   A. second and third
   B. third and fourth
   C. third, fourth, and fifth
   D. fourth and sixth
   E. fourth and fifth

7. Muscle elements in the second pair of pharyngeal arches give rise to which of the following muscles?
   A. frontal
   B. platysma
   C. orbicularis oculi
   D. buccinator
   E. all of the above

8. Which of the following cranial nerves supplies muscles derived from the first pair of pharyngeal arches?
   A. vagus
   B. glossopharyngeal
   C. facial
   D. trigeminal
   E. optic

9. How many *well-defined* pairs of human pharyngeal pouches develop?
   A. two
   B. three
   C. four
   D. five
   E. six

10. Structures derived from the first pharyngeal pouch include
    A. tympanic antrum
    B. tympanic cavity
    C. tubotympanic recess
    D. pharyngotympanic tube
    E. all of the above

11. The most common congenital anomaly of the head and neck is
    A. cleft palate
    B. bilateral cleft lip
    C. oblique facial cleft
    D. unilateral cleft lip
    E. median cleft lip

12. Which of the following structures is derived from the fourth pair of pharyngeal pouches?
    A. thymic corpuscles
    B. superior parathyroid glands
    C. inferior parathyroid glands
    D. thymus
    E. thyroid gland

13. An infant had a small blind sinus on the side of the neck along the anterior border of the sternocleidomastoid muscle. Mucus dripped intermittently from its opening. What is the most likely embryological basis of this congenital anomaly? Persistence of the embryonic opening of the
    A. second pharyngeal pouch
    B. second pouch and groove
    C. third pharyngeal groove
    D. thyroglossal duct
    E. second groove and cervical sinus

14. Cleft lip, with or without cleft palate, is common (about once in 1000 births). Which of the following is considered to be an important causative factor in the production of this anomaly?

A. riboflavin deficiency
B. infectious disease
C. mutant genes

D. cortisone
E. irradiation

15. The major portion of the human palate develops from the
    A. lateral palatine processes
    B. median palatine process
    C. intermaxillary segment
    D. medial nasal prominences
    E. frontonasal elevation

16. In DiGeorge syndrome, the development of the thymus and parathyroid glands are affected. Which of the following is involved?
    A. first pharyngeal pouch
    B. second pharyngeal pouch
    C. third pharyngeal pouch
    D. fourth pharyngeal pouch
    E. second and fourth pharyngeal pouches

17. When the palatine processes (shelves) fail to meet and fuse with each other and with the nasal septum, the resulting anomaly is a cleft of the
    A. uvula
    B. primary palate
    C. secondary palate
    D. intermaxillary segment
    E. primary and secondary palates

18. The greater horn and inferior part of the hyoid bone were absent in a 10-month-old infant. Which of the following embryonic structures was affected?
    A. maxillary prominence
    B. mandibular prominence
    C. second pharyngeal arch
    D. third pharyngeal arch
    E. fourth pharyngeal arch

19. Which of the following statements about the developing face is correct?
    A. Unilateral cleft lip results from failure of the medial nasal prominences to merge with each other.
    B. The nasolacrimal duct develops in a groove between the maxillary and lateral nasal prominences.
    C. The intermaxillary segment of the upper jaw is formed when the maxillary prominences merge with one another.
    D. Cleft lip, with or without cleft palate; occurs more frequently in females.
    E. The lower part of the face develops from the maxillary prominences.

20. With respect to the development of the palate, each of the following is correct *except:*
    A. If both lateral palatine processes fuse with the median palatine process but fail to fuse with the nasal septum and each other, a bilateral cleft of the secondary palate results.
    B. The palatine processes are derived from the maxillary and merged medial nasal prominences.
    C. Ossification of the palate does not extend posterior to the nasal septum.
    D. Fusion of the lateral palatine processes with each other begins in the sixth week.
    E. The primary palate develops from the intermaxillary segment of the maxilla.

21. The external acoustic meatus develops from the
    A. first pharyngeal groove
    B. second pharyngeal groove
    C. first pharyngeal pouch
    D. second pharyngeal pouch
    E. first pharyngeal groove and pouch

22. Concerning cleft of the upper lip, which of the following statements are correct?
    A. The incidence is about 1:2500 live births.
    B. Cleft lip occurs more frequently in females than males.
    C. Cleft lip results from failure of fusion/merging between the maxillary prominence and the merged medial nasal prominences.
    D. Cleft lip is embryologically indistinct from cleft palate.
    E. Median cleft lip is more common than bilateral cleft lip.

23. An infant was diagnosed as having a primary cleft of the palate. This congenital defect is
    A. located anterior to the incisive fossa
    B. caused by failure of the lateral palatine processes to meet and fuse in the midline.
    C. located lateral to the incisive fossa
    D. more common in males than in females
    E. due to the absence of lateral palatal shelves

24. A 30-year-old woman visited her doctor because of a painless swelling on the right side of her neck. A CT scan revealed a well-defined cystic mass at the angle of the mandible, just anterior to the sternocleidomastoid muscle. The most likely diagnosis is
    A. lateral cervical cyst
    B. thyroglossal duct cyst
    C. dermoid cyst
    D. swollen lymph node
    E. accessory thyroid tissue

## Answers and Explanations

1. **E** Pharyngeal arches, grooves, membranes and pouches are parts of the human pharyngeal apparatus that develops during the fourth week. This apparatus subsequently is transformed into various structures in the head and neck. For example, the pharyngeal pouches are modified to form structures like the tympanic cavity and the parathyroid glands.

2. **E** The cartilages of the third pair of pharyngeal arches give rise to the greater horns of the hyoid bone and to the inferior part of the body of this bone. The lesser horns and the superior part of the body of the hyoid bone are derived from the second pharyngeal arch cartilages.

3. **B** The facial nerve (CN/VII) is not a component of the first pharyngeal arch; it is the nerve of the second arch. The nerve of the first arch is the trigeminal nerve (CN V). The malleus is derived from the dorsal end of the first arch cartilage. The mandibular prominence is the larger of the two prominences of the first arch; it forms one side of the mandible. The maxillary prominence of the first arch, smaller than the mandibular prominence, contributes to the maxilla. Meckel cartilage is the eponymous name often given to the first arch cartilage; it gives rise to two middle ear bones (malleus and incus), but the mandible forms by intramembranous bone formation around the first arch cartilage as it degenerates.

4. **A** The incus is not derived from the second pharyngeal arch cartilage. It is formed by endochondral ossification of the dorsal end of the first arch cartilage (Meckel cartilage). In addition to the derivatives of the second arch cartilage listed, the stylohyoid ligament is derived from its perichondrium.

5. **B** The first and second pairs of pharyngeal arches are visible on each side of the future head and neck region by about 24 days. The third pair is recognizable by 26 days, and four pairs are present by the end of the fourth week. The fifth and sixth pairs of arches are rudimentary and are not recognizable externally.

6. **D** The thyroid, cricoid, arytenoid, corniculate, and cuneiform cartilages are derived mainly from the fused cartilages of the fourth and sixth arch cartilages. The fifth pharyngeal arch is rudimentary and soon degenerates. Often it does not develop. The cartilage in the epiglottis develops later than the other cartilages from mesenchyme derived from the hypopharyngeal (hypobranchial) eminence, a derivative of the third and fourth pair of pharyngeal arches.

7. **E** All these muscles are derived from myoblasts that differentiate from mesenchyme in the second pair of pharyngeal arches. During development, some myoblasts from the second arch migrate into the head, mainly to the facial region, and give rise to the muscles of facial expression. During their extensive migration, the developing muscles take their nerve supply (facial nerve) with them from the second arch.

8. **D** The fifth cranial nerve (trigeminal nerve) supplies the muscles of mastication and other muscles derived from myoblasts in the first pharyngeal arch. Because mesenchyme from the arches also contributes to the dermis and mucous membranes of the head and neck, these areas are supplied with sensory or branchial afferent fibers in the same nerve. The ophthalmic division of CN V does not supply arch derivatives.

9. **C** There are four well-defined pairs of pharyngeal pouches. The fifth pair is rudimentary or does not form; if present, they either disappear or are incorporated into the fourth pharyngeal pair of pouches to form the so-called caudal pharyngeal complex.

10. **E** All these structures are derived from the first pharyngeal pouch. The pouch expands into an elongate, tubotympanic recess that envelops the middle ear bones (auditory ossicles) derived from the dorsal ends of the first and second arch cartilages. The stalk of the recess gives rise to the lining of the pharyngotympanic (auditory) tube, and the expanded distal part becomes the lining of the tympanic cavity and antrum of the middle ear.

11. **D** Cleft lip, with or without cleft palate, occurs in about 1:1000 births. Unilateral cleft lip is more common than bilateral cleft lip. Cleft palate, with or without cleft lip, occurs in about 1:2500 births. Median cleft lip and oblique facial clefts are uncommon congenital anomalies. Cleft lip and cleft palate are embryologically and etiologically distinct anomalies.

12. **B** The superior parathyroid glands are derived from the fourth pair of pharyngeal pouches. One would think that the superior parathyroid glands would be derived from the third rather than the fourth pair of pouches. The reason they are not is that the parathyroids from the third pair of pharyngeal pouches are attached to the thymus and descend with it to a more inferior level than the parathyroids derived from the fourth pair of pouches.

13. **E** The anomaly probably is a lateral cervical sinus, resulting from the persistence of the opening into the cervical sinus. During the fifth week, the second pharyngeal arch grows over the third and fourth arches, forming an ectodermal depression — the cervical sinus. The second pharyngeal groove and the opening into the cervical sinus normally are obliterated as the neck forms. If the opening persists, it usually appears as an external pit or sinus on the side of the inferior one-third of the neck.

14. **C** Cleft lip in animals appears to have a mixed genetic and environmental causation, but practically nothing is known about environmental factors that may be involved in the production of this defect in human embryos. Experimental work in mice has consistently shown that cortisone causes cleft palate in a high incidence of fetuses, but it is not known to cause cleft lip in mouse or human embryos. Studies in humans indicate that genetic factors are of more importance in cleft lip, with or without cleft palate, than in cleft palate alone. If the parents are normal and have one child with a cleft lip, the chance that the next child will have a cleft lip is 4%. If one of the parents has cleft lip and they have a child with a cleft lip, the probability that the next child will be affected is 17%. Thus, mutant genes appear to be the important causative factors.

15. **A** The lateral palatine processes (shelves) of the maxillary prominences of the first pair

of pharyngeal arches give rise to the posterior or secondary palate. The primary palate or median palatine process develops from the innermost portion of the intermaxillary segment of the upper jaw. This segment, derived from the merged medial nasal prominences, gives rise to the small premaxillary region of the palate.

16. **C** In DiGeorge syndrome, the thymus and parathyroid glands are absent. Other anomalies are also present. The thymus develops from endoderm of the third pair of pharyngeal pouches and the surrounding mesenchyme. Recent experimental studies indicate that cells of neural crest origin are also involved in the development of the thymus.

17. **C** Clefts of the posterior or secondary palate result from failure of mesenchymal masses in the lateral palatine processes to meet and fuse with each other and the nasal septum. Such clefts extend through the soft and hard parts of the palate and are located posterior to the incisive fossa. Clefts anterior to the incisive fossa are clefts of the anterior or primary palate and result from a deficiency of mesenchyme in the maxillary prominence(s) and the intermaxillary segment.

18. **D** The cartilage of the third pharyngeal arch ossifies to form the greater horn (cornu) and the inferior part of the hyoid bone. The other derivative of this pharyngeal arch is the stylopharyngeus muscle.

19. **B** The nasolacrimal duct develops from a cord-like thickening of ectoderm in the floor of the groove between the maxillary and lateral nasal prominences. Failure of the cordlike thickening of ectoderm to canalize results in atresia of the nasolacrimal duct, the most common disorder of the lacrimal apparatus.

20. **D** The primary palate develops from the deep part of the intermaxillary segment of the maxilla (merged medial nasal prominences). It represents a relatively small part of the adult hard palate. The lateral palatine processes begin to develop in the sixth week from the maxillary prominences. Fusion of the lateral palatine processes with each other in the median plane,

and with the primary palate anteriorly, begins during the ninth week and is completed by the twelfth week.

21. **A** The external acoustic meatus (auditory canal) develops from the first pharyngeal groove. The remaining three pharyngeal grooves become obliterated by the second pharyngeal arch, which grows over them as the neck develops. The first pharyngeal pouch gives rise to the tympanic cavity, mastoid antrum, and pharyngotympanic tube.

22. **C** Clefting of the upper lip is a relatively common congenital anomaly with an incidence of about 1:1000 live births. It occurs more commonly in males. Cleft lip may be unilateral or bilateral and results from a failure of the maxillary prominence to merge with the medial nasal prominence. Although cleft lip and cleft palate frequently occur together, the embryological basis of cleft lip is distinct from that of cleft palate. Median cleft lip is very uncommon in humans.

23. **A** Failure of the lateral palatine processes to fuse with the primary palate results in a primary cleft palate (anterior cleft anomaly). It is located anterior to the incisive fossa. When the lateral palatine processes fail to meet and fuse in the midline, the resulting condition is described as a posterior cleft anomaly. This defect is located posterior to the incisive fossa, and occurs more commonly in females.

24. **A** The first pharyngeal groove gives rise to the external acoustic meatus. The remaining three (second, third, and fourth) pharyngeal grooves normally become obliterated by the second pharyngeal arch, which overgrows them. A transient ectoderm-lined cervical sinus is formed, which may persist as a lateral cervical or branchial cyst. The cervical cyst is usually located at the angle of the mandible, anterior to the sternocleidomastoid muscle. It may appear at any age, but it usually appears in young adults. Accessory thyroid tissue, thyroglossal duct cyst, and dermoid cyst are found in the midline of the neck. They usually are diagnosed at birth or within the first few years of life. The CT scan observations indicate that the diagnosis of a swollen lymph node is not present.

# Five-Choice Association Questions

**Directions:** Each group of questions below consists of a numbered list of descriptive words or phrases accompanied by a diagram with certain parts indicated by letters or by a list of lettered headings. For each numbered word or phrase, **select the lettered part or heading** that matches it correctly and then insert the letter in the space to the right of the appropriate number. Sometimes more than one numbered word or phrase may be correctly matched to the same lettered part or heading.

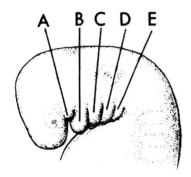

1. _____ Supplied by vagus nerve
2. _____ Its cartilage forms stapes
3. _____ Forms inferior part of face
4. _____ Gives rise to lateral palatine process
5. _____ Its muscle element gives rise to platysma
6. _____ Its cartilage forms a greater horn of hyoid bone

A. First pharyngeal arch
B. Second pharyngeal arch
C. Third pharyngeal arch

D. Fourth pharyngeal arch
E. Sixth pharyngeal arch

7. _____ Glossopharyngeal nerve
8. _____ Muscles of facial expression
9. _____ Supplied by maxillary division of fifth cranial nerve
10. _____ Stylohyoid ligament
11. _____ Superior laryngeal branch of vagus nerve
12. _____ Mandibular cartilage
13. _____ Gives rise to lateral palatine process
14. _____ Greater horn of hyoid bone
15. _____ Forms lateral part of upper lip
16. _____ Lesser horns of hyoid bone
17. _____ Main contributor to thyroid cartilage
18. _____ Supplied by CN X

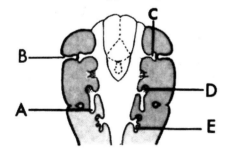

19. _____ Becomes external acoustic meatus
20. _____ Forms inferior parathyroid gland
21. _____ Tubotympanic recess
22. _____ Gives rise to ultimopharyngeal body
23. _____ Forms half of thymus
24. _____ Gives rise to pharyngotympanic tube

A. First pharyngeal pouch
B. Second pharyngeal pouch
C. Third pharyngeal pouch

D. Fourth pharyngeal pouch
E. Fifth pharyngeal pouch

25. _____ Thymus
26. _____ Superior parathyroid gland
27. _____ Inferior parathyroid gland
28. _____ May not develop

29. _____ Palatine tonsil
30. _____ Tubotympanic recess
31. _____ Internal branchial sinus
32. _____ Calcitonin

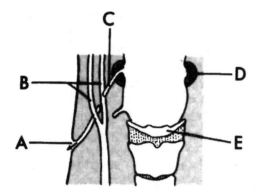

33. _____ Derived from second and third pharyngeal arch cartilages
34. _____ Internal branchial sinus
35. _____ Derived from second pharyngeal groove and cervical sinus
36. _____ External branchial sinus
37. _____ Internal and external carotid arteries
38. _____ Organ derived from second pharyngeal pouch and mesenchyme

## Answers and Explanations

1. **E** The fourth pharyngeal arch is supplied by the superior laryngeal branch of the vagus nerve (CN X). This nerve supplies pharyngeal and laryngeal muscles that develop from this arch.

2. **C** The dorsal end of the second arch cartilage (Reichert cartilage) ossifies to form the stapes of the middle ear and the styloid process of the temporal bone. The ventral ends of the cartilages form the lesser horns and the superior part of the body of the hyoid bone. The perichondrium of this cartilage forms the stylohyoid ligament.

3. **B** The mandibular prominences of the first pharyngeal arches form the inferior part of the face. The mandible develops in these prominences by intramembranous bone formation around the first arch cartilages.

4. **A** The lateral palatine processes arise as mesenchymal projections from the inner surfaces of the maxillary prominences of the first pharyngeal arches. The lateral palatine processes grow toward each other and fuse to form the posterior palate.

5. **C** The muscle elements in the second pair of pharyngeal arches give rise to myoblasts that migrate into the facial region and around the ears and eyes. These myoblasts differentiate into the muscles of facial expression.

6. **D** The third arch cartilages, located in the ventral portions of the arches, ossify to form the greater horns (cornua) and the inferior part of the body of the hyoid bone.

7. **C** The glossopharyngeal nerve (CN IX) is the nerve of the third pharyngeal arch; it supplies the stylopharyngeus muscle derived from the muscle element in this arch. Because the dorsal part of the root of the tongue is derived from the third arch, its sensory innervation is partly supplied by the glossopharyngeal nerve.

8. **B** The muscles of facial expression are derived from the second pharyngeal arch. Other muscles derived from this arch are the stylohyoid, posterior belly of digastric, and stapedius. From the position of the second arch in the embryo, one would not expect it to give rise to facial muscles. During development, the primordial muscle cells (myoblasts) migrate to the head and retain their original nerve supply from the second arch (i.e., the facial nerve).

9. **A** The maxillary prominence of the first pharyngeal arch is supplied by the maxillary division of the trigeminal nerve (CN $V_2$). The mandibular prominence is supplied by the mandibular branch of this nerve (CN $V_3$). The trigeminal nerve also supplies the muscles of mastication and other muscles derived from this arch. This nerve also supplies the skin over the mandible and the anterior two-thirds of the tongue.

10. **B** The stylohyoid ligament is derived from the perichondrium of the second pharyngeal arch cartilage, after it regresses between the styloid process and hyoid bone.

11. **D** The superior laryngeal branch of the vagus nerve (CN X) supplies the fourth pharyngeal

arch. Hence, it supplies the cricothyroid muscle and the constrictors of the pharynx that are derived from the muscle element in this arch.

12. **B**   The mandibular cartilage is the cartilage in the mandibular process of the first pharyngeal arch. Its dorsal portion, related to the developing internal ear, becomes ossified to form two middle ear bones (malleus and incus). The eponymous terms for the second arch cartilage is Meckel cartilage.

13. **A**   The maxillary prominences of the first pair of pharyngeal arches give rise to two internal projections — lateral palatine processes. These processes later fuse with each other and with the nasal septum to form the posterior or secondary palate. Incomplete fusion of these processes results in a cleft of the posterior palate.

14. **C**   The greater horns of the hyoid bone are derived from the cartilages of the third pair of pharyngeal arches. The inferior part of the body of this bone is also derived by endochondral ossification of these cartilages.

15. **A**   The maxillary prominence of the first pharyngeal arch gives rise to the lateral part of the upper lip. It fuses with the intermaxillary segment (merged medial nasal prominences), which forms the central portion or philtrum of the lip.

16. **B**   The lesser horns of the hyoid bone are derived from the cartilages of the second pharyngeal arches. The superior part of the body of this bone is also derived by endochondral ossification of these cartilages.

17. **D**   The cartilages of the fourth pair of pharyngeal arches give rise to large parts of the thyroid cartilage. The cartilages of the sixth arches also contribute to the laryngeal cartilages.

18. **D**   The fourth pharyngeal arch is supplied by the vagus nerve (CN X). This nerve supplies the intrinsic muscles of the larynx, which develop from myoblasts in this arch.

19. **B**   The external acoustic meatus develops from the dorsal end of the first pharyngeal groove.

All other pharyngeal grooves normally disappear as the neck forms.

20. **D**   The solid dorsal bulbar portion of the third pharyngeal pouch differentiates into an inferior parathyroid gland. These glands descend with the thymus gland and later leave it to lie on the posterior surface of the thyroid gland.

21. **C**   The tubotympanic recess becomes the pharyngotympanic tube, tympanic cavity, and antrum. Its epithelium forms the internal layer of the tympanic membrane.

22. **E**   The ventral portions of the fourth pharyngeal pouch give rise to the ultimopharyngeal body. If present, the fifth pair of pouches may also contribute to the formation of these bodies. The ultimopharyngeal bodies later fuse with the thyroid gland and are represented by cells called C or parafollicular cells. These cells produce calcitonin, an important hormone concerned with calcium metabolism.

23. **A**   The ventral portions of the third pair of pharyngeal pouches fuse and give rise to the primordium of the thymus. This thymic mass is invaded by mesenchymal cells that break up the gland into lobules. The thymic corpuscles (Hassall corpuscles) appear to be derived from the endodermal epithelium. The origin of the thymocytes is controversial, but they are believed to be mesenchymal.

24. **C**   The tubotympanic recess gives rise to the epithelium and glands of the pharyngotympanic tube. The bony wall in its posterior third and the remaining cartilaginous wall are derived from the surrounding mesenchyme.

25. **C**   The elongated ventral parts of the third pair of pharyngeal pouches migrate medially and fuse to form the primordium of the thymus. Development of the thymus is not complete at birth; it continues to grow and reaches its greatest size at puberty. Thereafter it becomes very small and is difficult to locate.

26. **D**   The dorsal bulbar part of each fourth pharyngeal pouch develops into a superior parathyroid gland. They come to lie on the dorsal surface of the thyroid gland.

27. **C**   The dorsal bulbar part of each third pharyngeal pouch differentiates into a parathyroid gland. These glands migrate caudally with the thymus, which develops from the ventral portions of this pair of pharyngeal pouches. Hence, the parathyroid glands derived from the third pair of pouches come to lie further caudally than those from the fourth pair of pouches. Because of this descent, sometimes the inferior parathyroid glands are located in other than their normal position; that is, they may be drawn into the thorax by the descent of the thymus.

28. **E**   The fifth pair of pharyngeal pouches may not develop. When present, they are rudimentary and incorporated into the fourth pair of pharyngeal pouches.

29. **B**   The palatine tonsils are derived from the endoderm of the second pair of pharyngeal pouches and the associated mesenchyme. The endoderm of the pouches gives rise to the surface epithelium and the lining of the crypts of the tonsil. The mesenchyme around the developing crypts differentiates into lymphoid tissue.

30. **A**   The epithelium and the glands of the pharyngotympanic tube are derived from the elongated tubotympanic recess, the expanded first pharyngeal pouch. This recess also gives rise to the tympanic cavity and antrum. The connective tissue and cartilaginous parts of the tube are derived from the mesenchyme surrounding the tubotympanic recess.

31. **B**   Internal branchial sinuses open into the pharynx. They commonly are derived from a remnant of the second pharyngeal pouch; hence, they typically open into the intratonsillar fossa, the remains of the opening into the second pharyngeal pouch.

32. **D**   Calcitonin is produced by the parafollicular cells (C cells) of the thyroid gland, derived from the ultimopharyngeal bodies. These bodies develop from the ventral portions of the fourth pair of pharyngeal pouches. If the fifth pair of pouches develop, they may contribute to the formation of the ultimobranchial bodies.

33. **E**   The hyoid bone develops by endochondral ossification of the ventral ends of the second and third pharyngeal arch cartilages. The second arch cartilages give rise to the lesser cornua and the superior part of the body, and the third arch cartilages give rise to the greater cornua and the inferior part of the body of the hyoid bone.

34. **C**   Internal branchial sinuses opening into the pharynx are uncommon. Because they almost always open into the intratonsillar fossa or near the palatopharyngeal arch, these sinuses usually result from partial persistence of part of the second pharyngeal pouch. These pouches commonly give rise to the epithelium and the lining of the crypts of the palatine tonsils.

35. **A**   External branchial sinuses (lateral cervical sinuses) are uncommon. Almost all of those that open on the side of the neck result from failure of the second pharyngeal groove to obliterate. The sinuses typically open on the inferior one third of a line that runs from the auricle of the ear along the anterior border of the sternocleidomastoid muscle to the jugular notch. There often is an intermittent discharge of mucus from the opening, resulting from infection of the sinus.

36. **A**   External branchial (lateral cervical) sinuses are lined with stratified squamous or columnar epithelium; they are surrounded by a muscular wall. Thus, by pulling the skin inferiorly, it is possible to palpate the firm sinus as it extends superiorly.

37. **B**   Sinuses and fistulas ascend through the subcutaneous tissue and the platysma muscle and between the external and internal carotid arteries.

38. **D**   The surface epithelium and lining of the crypts of the palatine tonsils are derived from the endoderm of the second pair of pharyngeal pouches. The mesenchyme that surrounds the pouches differentiates into lymphoid tissue that soon becomes organized into lymph nodules.

# Respiratory System

**11**

## Objectives

Be able to:

- Describe the early development of the lower respiratory system, illustrating the formation of the laryngotracheal tube and its derivatives.
- List the four stages of lung development, and discuss the main events that occur during each period.
- Write a brief note on surfactant and the respiratory distress syndrome.
- Discuss and illustrate the embryological basis of tracheoesophageal fistula with esophageal atresia.

## Five-Choice Completion Questions

**Directions:** Each of the following statements or questions is followed by five suggested responses or completions. **Select the one best answer** in each case.

1. The first indication of the lower respiratory tract in the human embryo is the laryngotracheal groove. It begins to develop in the primordial pharyngeal floor at _____ days.
   A. 19 to 21
   B. 22 to 24
   C. 25 to 27
   D. 28 to 30
   E. 31 to 33

2. The connective tissue, cartilage, and smooth muscle of the trachea are derived from the
   A. somatic mesoderm from the lateral plates
   B. splanchnic mesenchyme around the laryngotracheal tube
   C. endodermal lining of the laryngotracheal tube
   D. mesenchyme from the fourth to sixth pairs of pharyngeal arches
   E. neural crest

3. One-eighth to one-sixth of the adult number of alveoli are present in the lungs at birth. Their number increases after birth for at least _____ years.
   A. 2
   B. 4
   C. 6
   D. 8
   E. 10

4. A male infant showed signs of difficulty in breathing and his abdomen was distended. A common lower respiratory tract anomaly was diagnosed. Which of the following anomalies of the lower respiratory tract is most common?
   A. tracheal stenosis
   B. tracheal diverticulum
   C. tracheal atresia
   D. congenital emphysema
   E. tracheoesophageal fistula

5. Pulmonary surfactant is produced by
   A. alveolar epithelial cells
   B. blood cells
   C. alveolar macrophages (phagocytes)
   D. endothelial cells
   E. type II alveolar epithelial cells

6. Pulmonary surfactant begins to form in the human fetus at about _____ weeks.
   A. 16
   B. 20
   C. 24
   D. 28
   E. 32

7. A fetus born prematurely during which of the following periods of lung development may survive?
   A. organogenetic
   B. terminal sac
   C. pseudoglandular
   D. canalicular
   E. embryonic

8. The lungs at birth are about half inflated with liquid derived largely from the
   A. lung tissues
   B. nasal mucus
   C. amniotic fluid
   D. tracheal glands
   E. maternal blood

9. Hyaline membrane disease was suspected in a premature infant who showed signs of labored breathing and tachypnea at birth. This condition is caused by which of the following?
   A. deficiency of pulmonary surfactant
   B. excess pulmonary surfactant
   C. abnormal differentiation of type I alveolar cells
   D. intrauterine asphyxia
   E. atelectasis

10. Radiographic examination of an infant's lungs revealed areas of increased parenchymal density. A diagnosis of congenital lung cysts was made. The embryological basis of this defect involves which of the following?
    A. hypoplasia of the lungs
    B. deficiency of surfactant
    C. dilation of terminal bronchi
    D. defective tracheoesophageal septum
    E. tracheal atresia

11. A large mass of nonfunctional lung tissue was seen in the chest radiograph of a young girl. A diagnosis of pulmonary sequestration (accessory lung tissue) was made. This condition is probably due to
    A. failure of a bronchial bud to develop
    B. deficiency of pulmonary surfactant
    C. disturbance in bronchial tree development
    D. a fistula between the trachea and esophagus
    E. abnormal formation of an accessory lung bud

12. Fetal breathing movements
    A. occur regularly and continuously
    B. facilitate exchange of oxygen and carbon dioxide between mother and fetus
    C. decrease as the time of delivery approaches
    D. are essential for fetal lung development
    E. prevent aspiration of amniotic fluid

13. A newborn infant was observed to have continuous coughing and choking. There was an excessive amount of mucous secretion and saliva in the infant's mouth. The infant showed considerable diffculty in breathing. The physician was not able to pass a catheter through the esophagus into the stomach. The most likely diagnosis is
    A. tracheal stenosis
    B. tracheal atresia
    C. hyaline membrane disease
    D. duodenal atresia
    E. esophageal atresia with tracheoesophageal fistula

## Answers and Explanations

1. **C** The median longitudinal laryngotracheal groove is recognizable at 26 to 27 days. As it deepens, its caudal end begins to separate from the foregut, giving rise to the tracheal and esophageal primordia. This division extends cranially until only the communication between the pharynx and the air passages (the laryngeal inlet) remains.

2. **B** The connective tissue, cartilage, and smooth muscle of the trachea and bronchi develop from splanchnic mesenchyme around the laryngotracheal tube. The striated muscles, cartilages, and connective tissues of the larynx are derived from mesenchyme of the fourth to sixth pairs of branchial arches.

3. **D** Alveolar production begins in the human lungs during the late fetal period, but characteristic pulmonary alveoli probably do not form until respiration begins. Alveoli continue to form until at least the eighth year. About 30 to 50 million alveoli are present at birth, and by the eighth year, about 300 million alveoli are present. The number of alveoli in the adult lung varies between 250 and 500 million.

4. **E** Tracheoesophageal fistula occurs about once in 2500 births, predominantly in males. This connection between the trachea and esophagus results from incomplete separation of the respiratory and digestive portions of the foregut. In most cases, there is also esophageal atresia. The other listed anomalies occur less frequently.

5. **E** The type II alveolar epithelial cells produce surfactant, a surface-active agent. Surfactant forms a monomolecular layer over pulmonary alveolar surfaces and is capable of lowering surface tension at the air-alveolar interface when respiration begins at birth, thereby maintaining patency of the alveoli. Absence or deficiency of surfactant is a major cause of hyaline membrane disease.

6. **C** The type II cells of the epithelium of the alveoli, or secretory cells, begin to produce surfactant at about 24 weeks. It has been suggested that prolonged intrauterine asphyxia may produce reversible changes in these cells, making them incapable of producing surfactant. However, there are probably several causes for absence or deficiency of surfactant, particularly in premature infants.

7. **B** During the terminal sac period (24 weeks to birth), a fetus may survive if born prematurely, especially if it weighs 1000 gm or more. The terminal air sacs appear as outpouchings of the respiratory bronchioles and are soon surrounded by a rich capillary network. Before this time, the fetal lungs usually are incapable of providing adequate gas exchange, mainly because of inadequate pulmonary vasculature.

8. **A** The fluid in the lungs at birth is believed to be derived mainly from the lower respiratory tract itself. As much as 30 ml/day of fluid may be produced by the fetal tracheobronchial tree near term. The fluid in the lungs differs in composition from plasma, lymph, and amniotic fluid. Some of the liquid in the lungs probably comes from the tracheal glands, and some is

probably amniotic fluid. It is well established that respiratory movements occur before birth, causing aspiration of amniotic fluid.

9. **A** Pulmonary surfactant, produced by type II alveolar cells, counteracts surface tension forces and facilitates expansion of the terminal sacs or primordial alveoli. Surfactant deficiency leads to hyaline membrane disease, a common cause of neonatal deaths, especially among infants born prematurely.

10. **C** Congenital lung cysts arise from abnormal development and dilation of the terminal bronchi. Because of air or fluid in the cysts, the lungs have a honeycomb appearance on radiographs.

11. **E** Pulmonary sequestration (accessory lung tissue) is an aberrant mass of nonfunctional lung tissue that does not communicate with the tracheobronchial tree. It is believed that pulmonary sequestration, intralobular (in the lung) or extralobular (outside the lung), results from abnormal development of an accessory lung bud derived from the foregut of the embryo. This nonfunctional mass of pulmonary tissue is nourished by systemic arteries. Pulmonary sequestration is usually detected as an incidental finding on chest radiography or at surgery, and most are resected. Deficiency of pulmonary surfactant is associated with hyaline membrane disease. Failure of a bronchial bud to develop leads to agenesis of a lung. Tracheo-esophageal fistula results from incomplete separation of the trachea and the esophagus during their development from the foregut.

12. **D** Periodic breathing movements occur in utero and cause aspiration of amniotic fluid into the lungs. Exchange of gases between mother and fetus occurs in the placenta before birth and in the lungs after birth. The fluid in the lungs is cleared at birth and replaced by gases with the infant's breathing. Prenatal breathing movements stimulate lung development. Fetal breathing movements can be detected and monitored by real-time ultrasonography. The pattern of fetal breathing movements is used for diagnosis of labor and for assessing fetal outcome in preterm delivery.

13. **E** Esophageal atresia results from deviation of the tracheoesophageal septum in a posterior direction. It occurs in 3000 to 4500 live births and is often associated with tracheoesophageal fistula. The fetus is unable to swallow amniotic fluid which leads to polyhydramnios (accumulation of an excessive amount of amniotic fluid).

# Five-Choice Association Questions

**Directions:** Each group of questions below consists of a numbered list of descriptive words or phrases accompanied by a diagram with certain parts indicated by letters or by a list of lettered headings. For each numbered word or phrase, **select the lettered part or heading** that matches it correctly and then insert the letter in the space to the right of the appropriate number. Sometimes more than one numbered word or phrase may be correctly matched to the same lettered part or heading.

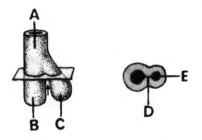

1. _____ Tracheal bud
2. _____ Esophagus
3. _____ Divides foregut into the laryngotracheal tube and esophagus
4. _____ Gives rise to the larynx, trachea, bronchi, and lungs
5. _____ Foregut
6. _____ Divides into bronchial buds

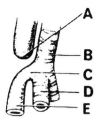

A. Laryngotracheal groove
B. Somatic mesoderm
C. Surfactant
D. Esophageal atresia
E. Splanchnic mesenchyme

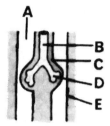

7. _____ Associated with polyhydramnios
8. _____ Derived from the tracheal bud
9. _____ Esophageal atresia
10. _____ Laryngotracheal fistula
11. _____ Allows air to enter the gastrointestinal tract

12. _____ Polyhydramnios
13. _____ Tracheal cartilage
14. _____ Type II alveolar cells
15. _____ Tracheoesophageal fistula
16. _____ Prevents atelectasis
17. _____ Diverticulum of pharynx
18. _____ Hyaline membrane disease
19. _____ Parietal pleura

20. _____ Primordium of the left lung
21. _____ Its glands are derived from the laryngotracheal tube
22. _____ Pericardioperitoneal canal
23. _____ Future right pleural cavity
24. _____ Splanchnic mesenchyme
25. _____ Forms parietal pleura

## *Answers and Explanations*

1. **C** The tracheal bud (lung bud) develops at the caudal end of the laryngotracheal tube and soon divides into two bronchial buds. These buds differentiate into the bronchi and their ramifications in the lungs.

2. **B** The esophagus is derived from the foregut and separated from the laryngotracheal tube when the tracheoesophageal septum formed.

3. **D** The tracheoesophageal septum, formed by the gradual fusion of the tracheoesophageal folds, divides the foregut into the laryngotracheal tube and the esophagus. Incomplete separation of these structures results in one of the varieties of tracheoesophageal fistula.

4. **E** The endodermal lining of the laryngotracheal tube gives rise to the epithelium and glands of the larynx, trachea, and bronchi and to the pulmonary lining epithelium. The connective tissue, cartilage, and smooth muscle of these structures develop from the surrounding splanchnic mesenchyme.

5. **A** The foregut gives rise to the pharynx and its derivatives, the lower respiratory tract, esophagus, stomach, and first part of the duodenum as far as the entry of the bile duct, and to the liver and pancreas.

6. **C** The tracheal bud that forms at the caudal end of the laryngotracheal tube during the fourth week gives rise to two bronchial buds. These buds differentiate into the bronchi and their ramifications in the lungs.

7. **A** Polyhydramnios (excess amniotic fluid) is frequent in mothers of fetuses that have esophageal atresia because amniotic fluid cannot pass to the intestines for absorption and subsequent transfer to the placenta for disposal. If you selected choice C, you were partly right because esophageal atresia often is associated

with tracheoesophageal fistula. Esophageal atresia may occur as a separate anomaly and tracheoesophageal fistula without esophageal atresia also occurs. With an isolated fistula, polyhydramnios probably would not be present because amniotic fluid could pass to the stomach and intestines.

8. **D**   The bronchi are derived from divisions of the tracheal bud called bronchial (lung) buds. These buds differentiate into the bronchi and their ramifications in the lungs.

9. **A**   Atresia or lack of continuity of the esophagus may be encountered as a separate congenital anomaly. Esophageal atresia commonly is associated with tracheoesophageal fistula. An overall incidence of these associated anomalies of 1:2500 neonates is accepted. About two thirds of the cases occur in males. Infants present with excessive saliva, gagging, vomiting if fed, and cyanosis. Aspiration of gastric contents is responsible for the severe pulmonary symptoms.

10. **C**   The type of tracheoesophageal fistula shown is the most common (more than 85% of cases). The fistula results from incomplete fusion of tracheoesophageal folds. This canal forms at the site of the defective tracheoesophageal septum and permits communication between the esophagus and trachea. The commonly associated esophageal atresia probably results from incomplete recanalization of the upper part of the esophagus.

11. **C**   In the usual type of tracheoesophageal fistula, associated with the inferior end of the esophageal atresia, there is a fistulous connection between the lower esophagus and the trachea (as shown). Not only does this fistula allow gastric contents to enter the lungs, causing severe pulmonary symptoms, but it permits air to enter the gastrointestinal tract. As a result, the abdomen rapidly becomes distended and the intestines promptly fill with air.

12. **D**   An excess of amniotic fluid commonly is associated with esophageal atresia and tracheoesophageal fistula because amniotic fluid cannot pass to the intestines for absorption and subsequent transfer to the placenta for dis-

posal. Polyhydramnios may also be associated with meroanencephaly (partial absence of the brain), possibly because the fetus lacks the neural control for swallowing amniotic fluid.

13. **E**   The tracheal cartilages develop from the splanchnic mesenchyme that surrounds the laryngotracheal tube. This mesenchyme also gives rise to the connective tissue and smooth muscle of the trachea.

14. **C**   Type II alveolar cells, the secretory cells of the lining epithelium, produce the surface-active agent called surfactant. These cells are believed to begin producing surfactant at about 24 weeks.

15. **D**   A tracheoesophageal fistula occurs about 1:2500 births, predominantly in males. In 85% of cases, this anomaly is associated with esophageal atresia.

16. **C**   Surfactant, a substance produced by the type II alveolar cells, is capable of lowering the surface tension at the air alveolar surface, thereby maintaining patency of the alveoli and preventing atelectasis (imperfect expansion or collapse of the lungs).

17. **A**   The longitudinal laryngotracheal groove is a diverticulum of the endodermal floor of the primordial pharynx, caudal to the hypopharyngeal eminence (primordium of the posterior one-third of the tongue and of the epiglottis). The endodermal lining of this groove gives rise to the epithelium and glands of the larynx, trachea, and bronchi and to the pulmonary lining epithelium.

18. **C**   Hyaline membrane disease, a common cause of death in the perinatal period, is associated with an absence or deficiency of surfactant. In this disease, which occurs particularly in babies born prematurely, a membrane-like structure lines the respiratory bronchioles, alveolar ducts, and alveoli. Because of the deficiency of surfactant, there is a tendency for the alveoli to collapse (atelectasis).

19. **B**   The parietal pleura develops from the mesoderm that lines the thoracic body wall. As the lungs invaginate the pericardioperitoneal cavities (primitive pleural cavities), the space

between the parietal and visceral layers of pleura is reduced to a narrow interval.

20. **D**  The left bronchial bud, together with the surrounding splanchnic mesenchyme, gives rise to the left lung. At the stage shown, the bronchial buds represent the two lobes of the left lung.

21. **B**  The endodermal lining of the middle part of the laryngotracheal tube gives rise to the epithelium and glands of the trachea. The cartilage, connective tissue, and smooth muscle are derived from the surrounding splanchnic mesenchyme.

22. **A**  The pericardioperitoneal canal connects the pericardial cavity and the peritoneal cavity during the fourth and fifth weeks. After division of the intraembryonic coelom into three separate cavities, these canals become the pleural cavities.

23. **A**  The future right pleural cavity is represented by the right pericardioperitoneal canal. The developing lungs grow into the splanchnic mesoderm of the medial walls of the pericardioperitoneal canals.

24. **C**  The splanchnic mesenchyme surrounding the developing lungs gives rise to the bronchial musculature and cartilaginous rings and to the pulmonary connective tissue and capillaries. The splanchnic mesenchyme also gives rise to the visceral pleura covering the lungs.

25. **E**  The pleural cavities are lined externally by a layer of somatic mesoderm; this layer subsequently becomes the parietal pleura. The invagination of the lungs into the developing pleural cavities is so complete that the space between the visceral and parietal layers of pleura becomes greatly reduced.

# Digestive System

**12**

## Objectives

Be able to:

- Construct and label diagrams illustrating the formation of the primordial gut by the incorporation of part of the yolk sac into the embryo.
- List the derivatives of the foregut.
- Describe the rotation of the stomach and formation of the omental bursa.
- Describe the development of the duodenum, liver, biliary apparatus, pancreas, and spleen.
- List the derivatives of the midgut, and illustrate herniation, rotation, reduction, and fixation of the intestines.
- Write brief notes on pyloric stenosis, omphalocele, incomplete rotation and volvulus of the midgut, intestinal stenosis and atresia, and ileal (Meckel) diverticulum.
- List the derivatives of the hindgut.
- Describe partitioning of the cloaca.
- Describe development of the anal canal, and write short notes on imperforate anus and anorectal agenesis with fistula.

## Five-Choice Completion Questions

**Directions:** Each of the following statements or questions is followed by five suggested responses or completions. **Select the one best answer** in each case.

1. As the stomach acquires its adult shape, it rotates around its longitudinal axis. Which of the following events does not result from this rotation?
    A. Ventral border of the stomach moves to the right.
    B. Dorsal border of the stomach moves to the left.
    C. Dorsal mesogastrium is carried to the left.
    D. Dorsal part of the stomach grows rapidly.
    E. Duodenum slowly rotates to the right.

2. Derivatives of the caudal part of the embryonic foregut are mainly supplied by which of the following arteries?
    A. superior mesenteric
    B. inferior mesenteric
    C. gastro-omental
    D. celiac
    E. right gastric

3. Ultrasound examination of a pregnant woman near term revealed that the small intestines of the fetus had herniated into the amniotic cavity and was floating in the amniotic fluid. The condition was diagnosed as gastroschisis, which results from faulty development of the

    A. head fold                 D. lateral folds

    B. tail fold                    E. amnion

    C. neural folds

4. Hematopoiesis begins in the liver during the _____ week.

    A. third                    D. sixth

    B. fourth                 E. seventh

    C. fifth

5. The most common type of anorectal anomaly is

    A. anal stenosis             D. anal agenesis

    B. ectopic anus            E. persistent anal membrane

    C. anorectal agenesis

6. The anal membrane usually ruptures at the end of the _____ week.

    A. fifth                    D. eighth

    B. sixth                  E. ninth

    C. seventh

7. Pyloric stenosis is characterized by vomiting, usually starting in the second or third week after birth. The narrowing of the pyloric lumen results primarily from

    A. hypertrophy of the longitudinal muscular layer

    B. a diaphragm-like narrowing of the pyloric lumen

    C. hypertrophy of the circular muscular layer

    D. persistence of the solid stage of pyloric development

    E. a so-called fetal vascular accident in the pylorus

8. The junction of the endodermal epithelium of the hindgut and the ectodermal epithelium of the proctodeum (anal pit) is believed to be indicated by the

    A. pectinate line            D. external sphincter

    B. levator ani muscle       E. superior ends of the anal columns

    C. anal white line

9. An incidental finding of an ileal (Meckel) diverticulum was made in a 12-year-old boy. This condition

    A. is an uncommon anomaly of the small intestine

    B. represents the remnants of the allantoic diverticulum

    C. is located near the duodenojejunal junction

    D. is located on the antimesenteric border of the ileum

    E. occurs more frequently in females

10. Anorectal agenesis is more common in males than in females and is usually associated with a rectourethral fistula. The embryological basis of the fistula is

    A. failure of the proctodeum to develop     D. abnormal partitioning of the cloaca

    B. agenesis of the urorectal septum        E. premature rupture of the anal membrane

    C. failure of fixation of the hindgut

11. A 3-week-old infant has a history of projectile vomiting. The vomitus did not contain bile. The child cried frequently and was constantly hungry but did not gain weight. Which of the following conditions would best account for these symptoms?

A. Meckel diverticulum
B. esophageal atresia
C. hypertrophic pyloric stenosis

D. duodenal atresia
E. tracheoesophageal fistula

12. Massive rectal bleeding was observed in an infant. The color of the blood ranged from bright to dark red. The child appeared to be free of pain. A diagnosis of Meckel diverticulum was made. This condition is associated with which of the following?
    A. remnant of the yolk stalk
    B. duplication of the intestine
    C. subhepatic cecum and appendix

    D. nonrotation of the midgut
    E. herniation of the intestines

13. Esophageal atresia was diagnosed in a newborn infant with symptoms of excessive salivation and almost instant vomiting of food. This congenital defect is associated with
    A. oligohydramnios
    B. anterior deviation of the tracheoesophageal septum

    C. polyhydramnios
    D. postmaturity
    E. tracheal stenosis

14. Recanalization of the esophagus occurs during the _____ week of development.
    A. fourth
    B. sixth
    C. eighth

    D. tenth
    E. twelfth

15. A 28-year-old man died from complications after abdominal surgery. The pathologists found about two liters of blood in the omental bursa. The omental bursa or lesser sac
    A. develops in the mesenchyme of the dorsal mesogastrium
    B. develops in the mesenchyme of the ventral mesentery
    C. is a closed pouch
    D. results from rotation of the midgut loop
    E. lies between the stomach and anterior abdominal wall

16. The ventral mesentery of the foregut gives rise to which of the following?
    A. lesser omentum
    B. falciform ligament
    C. visceral peritoneum of liver

    D. hepatogastric ligament
    E. all of the above

17. Extrahepatic biliary atresia was diagnosed in a newborn infant. Regarding this congenital defect, which of the following statements is correct?
    A. It results from degeneration of the cells occluding the biliary ducts (vacuolation).
    B. It occurs in about 1:1000 to 1:2500 live births.
    C. This is the most serious anomaly of the extrahepatic biliary system.
    D. Liver infection during early embryonic development may result in extrahepatic biliary atresia.
    E. The bile duct arises from the midgut segment of the primordial gut.

18. A 22-year-old woman was admitted to the surgical clinic with symptoms of acute appendicitis. The surgeon decided to do an emergency laparotomy. During the operation the appendix was found to be normal. Instead, an inflammed diverticulum was located 2 feet from the ileocecal junction on the ileum. This diverticulum is the persistent remnant of
    A. allantois
    B. yolk stalk
    C. urorectal septum

    D. neuroenteric canal
    E. midgut loop

19. A 15-year-old male was surgically treated for a strangulated indirect inguinal hernia. The surgeon noticed that the small intestine was located in the right half of the abdominal cavity and the large intestine on the left side. The cecum and appendix were suprapubic in position. Which of the following would cause this anomaly?
    A. nonrotation of the midgut
    B. reversed rotation of the midgut
    C. midgut volvulus
    D. mixed rotation of the midgut
    E. duplication of the intestine

20. Ultrasound examination of a 40-year-old pregnant woman at 30 weeks' gestation revealed that the duodenum of the fetus was completely occluded. The ultrasound scan showed
    A. an empty stomach
    B. a "double-bubble" sign
    C. distended esophagus
    D. absence of the gallbladder
    E. polyhydramnios

21. Acute appendicitis was diagnosed in a young man with severe lower abdominal pain. The appendix
    A. develops from the embryonic midgut
    B. develops from the embryonic hindgut
    C. is located anterior to the cecum
    D. arises from the mesenteric border of the gut
    E. is invariable in position

22. The regional differentiation of the digestive tract is regulated by expression of
    A. *bHLH* proteins (basic helix-loop-helix)
    B. *hox* genes (homeobox genes)
    C. *BMPs* (bone morphogenetic proteins)
    D. *Notch* (notch pathway)
    E. *Shh* (sonic hedgehog)

## Answers and Explanations

1. **D** Growth of the stomach occurs during rotation, but it does not result from it. The faster growth of the original dorsal part of the stomach forms the greater curvature of the stomach. Rotation of the stomach explains why the left vagus nerve supplies the anterior wall of the adult stomach and why the right vagus innervates its posterior wall. As the stomach rotates, the duodenal loop rotates to the right.

2. **D** The celiac trunk (artery) supplies derivatives of the caudal part of the embryonic foregut (e.g., the stomach). It arises from the anterior aspect of the aorta just inferior to the aortic hiatus. It divides into the left gastric, hepatic, and splenic arteries, which supply most of the foregut derivatives (inferior part of the esophagus, stomach, superior part of the duodenum, liver, pancreas, and biliary apparatus). If you chose **C** or **E**, you selected a correct answer because they supply some foregut derivatives. **D** is the best answer, however, because it provides the main blood supply to the caudal part of the foregut.

3. **D** Gastroschisis is a relatively common defect of the abdominal wall. It results from incomplete closure of the lateral body folds during the fourth week. The viscera (including the intestines) protrude into the amniotic cavity and are bathed by amniotic fluid.

4. **D** Hematopoiesis (blood formation) begins in the mesenchyme of the yolk sac and allantois during the third week, but it does not begin in the embryonic mesenchyme until early in the sixth week. Hematopoiesis occurs chiefly in the liver and spleen. Later, blood formation occurs in bone marrow and lymph nodes, in which sites it continues after birth.

5. **C** In most anorectal anomalies, the rectum ends superior to the anal canal and levator ani muscles. There usually is a fistulous connection

with the urethra in males and the vagina in females. These defects produce intestinal obstruction because the fistulas seldom provide an adequate escape for gas and meconium (dark green fecal material).

6. **C** The anal membrane usually ruptures at the end of the seventh week. Imperforate anus resulting from failure of the anal membrane to perforate is uncommon. This type of imperforate anus consists of a septal occlusion of an otherwise normal anal canal. Some form of imperforate anus, usually anorectal agenesis, occurs about once in 5000 births and is much more common in males than in females. The reason for this sex difference is not known.

7. **C** Pyloric stenosis is common, especially in males (about 1 in 150). The pylorus is elongated and thickened to as much as twice its usual size. Forceful peristaltic waves of the gastric wall may be observed. The cause of pyloric stenosis is unknown, but hereditary factors are certainly involved. An acquired factor also appears to be involved in the pathogenesis of this "tumor," but its nature is unknown.

8. **A** The former site of the anal membrane, and thus the junction of the hindgut and the proctodeum, is believed to be indicated by the irregular pectinate line (*pectin,* Latin for comb). The anal valves are attached along this line. Because of the different origins of the superior and inferior parts of the anal canal, the blood and nerve supply of the two parts differ. The inferior part of the anal canal, inferior to the pectinate line, is supplied by somatic sensory cutaneous fibers that respond immediately to painful stimuli, such as the prick of a needle. Thus, injection of a hemorrhoidal vein in the therapy of internal hemorrhoids is given superior to the pectinate line, where the mucosa is relatively insensitive to pain.

9. **D** Diverticula of the ileum, usually called Meckel diverticula, are always on the antimesenteric border of the ileum because they represent a persistent part of the yolk stalk (vitello-intestinal duct), which attaches to the ventral side of the midgut loop. If a Meckel diverticulum inverts, it may serve as a leading point for intussusception (inversion of the diverticulum and ileum into the lumen of the ileum). Bleeding of a diverticulum arises from the peptic ulcer in or adjacent to the ectopic gastric mucosa, usually at the neck of the diverticulum. Meckel diverticulum occurs three to five times more frequently in males than in females.

10. **D** The urorectal septum, a mesenchymal septum or wedge between the allantois and the hindgut, typically grows caudally and fuses with the cloacal membrane. This partition divides the cloaca into the rectum dorsally and the urogenital sinus ventrally. Failure of the lateral infoldings of the cloaca, produced by caudal extensions of the urorectal septum, to fuse completely at all levels results in communication between the rectum and the urogenital sinus. The urogenital sinus in males gives rise to the urinary bladder and almost all the urethra. Thus, the fistula connects the rectum with the bladder (rectourethral fistula). In females, the urogenital sinus also gives rise to the vagina; rectovaginal fistulas are most commonly associated with anorectal agenesis in females.

11. **C** Congenital hypertrophic pyloric stenosis involves an increase in the size of the circular muscle of the pylorus. This results in severe narrowing of the pyloric canal and obstruction to the passage of food. The infant expels the contents of the stomach with considerable (projectile) force. Males are affected more than females (5:1), and the cause is unknown. Blockage or atresia of the duodenum is associated with vomiting within a few hours of birth, and the vomitus usually contains bile.

12. **A** The remnant of the proximal part of the yolk stalk forms an ileal (Meckel) diverticulum. It is the most frequent anomaly of the gastrointestinal tract and three to five times more prevalent in males than in females. Inflammation of the diverticulum can mimic the symptoms of acute appendicitis. The heterotopic gastric mucosa in the wall of the diverticulum may also cause bleeding from peptic ulceration. Other complications of Meckel diverticulum may be related to its connection with the

umbilicus, leading to a volvulus or torsion of intestinal loops.

13. **C**　A fetus with esophageal atresia is unable to swallow amniotic fluid, resulting in an excess of amniotic fluid or polyhydramnios. In more than 85% of cases, esophageal atresia is associated with a tracheoesophageal fistula. This communication between the trachea and esophagus is formed because of incomplete fusion of the tracheoesophageal folds. During the division of the foregut to form the laryngotracheal tube and esophagus, the tracheoesophageal septum may deviate in a posterior direction, resulting in an esophageal atresia. About one third of affected infants are born prematurely.

14. **C**　In the early embryo, the epithelial lining of the esophagus proliferates and partly or completely obliterates its lumen. During the eighth week, recanalization of the esophagus normally occurs and establishes the continuity of its lumen. Some isolated cases of esophageal atresia have been associated with a failure of recanalization of the esophagus. This condition has been attributed to defective growth of endodermal cells. Incomplete recanalization of the esophagus during the eighth week may lead to stenosis of the esophagus.

15. **A**　The omental bursa develops from isolated clefts in the mesenchyme of the dorsal mesentery. These clefts coalesce, forming the primordium of the omental bursa. The omental bursa (lesser sac) communicates with the main part of the peritoneal cavity through a small opening, the omental (epiploic) foramen. The omental bursa is located between the stomach and the posterior body wall. The bursa permits the stomach to move freely as well as to change its size and shape.

16. **E**　The ventral mesentery of the foregut contributes to the formation of the lesser omentum (hepatogastric ligament), which passes from the liver to the lesser curvature of the stomach. The ventral mesentery also forms the falciform ligament, which is a fold of peritoneum extending from the liver to the ventral abdominal wall. The peritoneal covering of the liver is also derived from the ventral mesentery. The

bile duct lies in the free margin of the lesser omentum, and the umbilical vein traverses the free border of the falciform ligament. Clinically, it is important to know the location of the bile duct and the umbilical vein. The hepatic diverticulum and the ventral pancreatic bud arise from the caudal part of the foregut.

17. **C**　Extrahepatic biliary atresia is the most serious anomaly of the extrahepatic biliary system. It occurs in 1:10,000 to 1:15,000 live births. The extrahepatic biliary duct system is derived from the foregut and becomes occluded in the early embryo because of proliferation of endodermal cells. Later, it is canalized. Biliary atresia is an extremely serious birth defect that requires surgical correction (portoenterostomy). When biliary atresia cannot be corrected surgically, the child may die if a liver transplantation is not performed. The 5-year survival for such patients is about 70%. Surgical correction of atresia involving the distal portion of the extrahepatic duct has a better prognosis than atresia of the proximal or the entire extrahepatic duct system.

18. **B**　The diverticulum is the persistent remnant of the proximal part of the yolk stalk (vitellointestinal duct). See also answer to question 9.

19. **A**　Nonrotation of the midgut or left-sided colon is a relatively common anomaly. It results from a failure of the midgut loop to rotate as it reenters the abdomen. The condition is usually asymptomatic but twisting of the intestine (volvulus) may occur. In reversed rotation, the midgut loop rotates in a clockwise rather than counterclockwise direction.

20. **B**　A "double-bubble" sign in the fetus suggests that the duodenum is completely occluded (duodenal atresia). The "double-bubble" appearance is caused by a distended gas-filled stomach and duodenum. Because duodenal atresia prevents the normal absorption of amniotic fluid by the intestines, oligohydramnios occurs.

21. **A**　The appendix arises as a diverticulum (cecal swelling) from the antimesenteric border of the midgut loop. The position of the appendix is variable. In about 64% of people, it is located retrocecally. Rarely, the cecum adheres to the

inferior surface of the liver when it returns to the abdomen, resulting in a subhepatic appendix. This may present problems in the diagnosis of appendicitis and surgical removal of the appendix (appendectomy).

22. **B** *Hox* genes, expressed in the endoderm and surrounding mesenchyme, play an essential role in the regionalization of the gut. The other listed molecular pathways are not involved in this process.

# Five-Choice Association Questions

**Directions:** Each group of questions below consists of a numbered list of descriptive words or phrases accompanied by a diagram with certain parts indicated by letters or by a list of lettered headings. For each numbered word or phrase, **select the lettered part or heading** that matches it correctly and then insert the letter in the space to the right of the appropriate number. Sometimes more than one numbered word or phrase may be correctly matched to the same lettered part or heading.

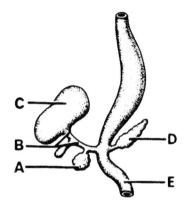

A. Spleen
B. Yolk stalk
C. Gallbladder
D. Appendix
E. Celiac trunk

1. _____ Primarily involved in extrahepatic biliary atresia
2. _____ Forms the major part of the pancreas
3. _____ Penetrates the septum transversum
4. _____ Partly derived from the midgut
5. _____ Forms the inferior part of the head of the pancreas
6. _____ Extends into the dorsal mesentery

7. _____ Derived from the midgut loop
8. _____ Continuous with the apex of the midgut loop
9. _____ Organ derived solely from mesenchyme
10. _____ Derived from foregut
11. _____ Supplies foregut derivatives
12. _____ Umbilical sinus

13. _____ Derived from the foregut and midgut
14. _____ Hepatoduodenal ligament
15. _____ Arises as a diverticulum of the foregut
16. _____ Visceral peritoneum
17. _____ Its free border contains umbilical vein
18. _____ Embryonic site of hematopoiesis

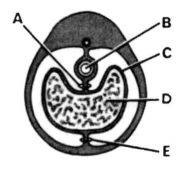

A. Pyloric stenosis
B. Anorectal agenesis
C. Esophageal atresia
D. Omphalocele
E. Polyhydramnios

19. _____ Faulty partitioning of foregut
20. _____ Herniation of intestines
21. _____ Causes projectile vomiting
22. _____ Duodenal obstruction
23. _____ Most common anomaly
24. _____ Faulty partitioning of cloaca

## Answers and Explanations

1. **B** In extrahepatic biliary atresia, parts of the hepatic ducts and bile duct are not canalized. Parts of the bile ducts are blocked (atresia); other parts may have narrow lumina (stenosis). These severe anomalies are not common. The extrahepatic system of bile ducts develops as solid cords that typically soon become canalized. When this fails to occur, atresia results. If the lumen forms but is small, stenosis is present. Congenital atresia of the bile ducts may be caused by noxious agents acting during the development of the bile duct system. There is little evidence that this anomaly is hereditary; it rarely occurs in siblings (brothers or sisters). Jaundice gradually increases after birth; the stools are clay-colored, and the urine is dark brown.

2. **D** The dorsal pancreatic bud forms the major part of the pancreas; the inferior part of the head of the pancreas and the uncinate process are derived from the ventral pancreatic bud. The main pancreatic duct forms by fusion of the ducts of both pancreatic buds.

3. **C** The liver arises as a bud from the caudal part of the foregut late in the third week. This hepatic diverticulum extends ventrally and cranially into the mesenchyme of the septum transversum between the pericardial cavity and the yolk stalk. Subsequently, the liver lies between the layers of the ventral mesentery. These layers become the peritoneal covering of the liver and the ligaments associated with the liver.

4. **E** The epithelium and glands of the duodenum distal to the point of entrance of the bile duct are derived from the midgut. Other layers of the mucous membrane and the wall of the duodenum are derived from mesenchyme adjacent to the endodermal midgut. The epithelium and glands of the duodenum cranial to the entrance of this duct are derived from the foregut.

5. **A** The ventral pancreatic bud forms the inferior part of the head of the pancreas, including the uncinate process. Most of the pancreas develops from the dorsal bud. Sometimes the two pancreatic buds form a ring of pancreatic tissue around the duodenum (anular pancreas), which may cause obstruction of the duodenum.

6. **D** The dorsal pancreatic bud from the caudal end of the foregut appears slightly before the ventral pancreatic bud. As it grows, it extends into the dorsal mesentery. During rotation and growth of the duodenum, the ventral bud is carried dorsally with the bile duct and, subsequently, fuses with the dorsal bud.

7. **D** The appendix is derived from the cecal diverticulum, an outpouching from the antimesenteric side of the midgut loop. The distal end of the cecum does not grow rapidly; thus, the appendix forms. At birth, the appendix is relatively longer than in the adult and continuous with the apex of the cecum.

8. **B** The yolk stalk is attached to the apex of the midgut loop. The other end of this stalk is attached to the remnant of the yolk sac, located near the placenta. The yolk stalk normally degenerates at the end of the embryonic period, but in about 2% of people, the proximal part of it persists as an ileal Meckel (diverticulum).

9. **A** The spleen is derived from a condensation of mesenchymal cells between the layers of the dorsal mesogastrium. The splenic artery is a branch of the foregut (celiac) artery; this explains why it gives off pancreatic branches, short gastric arteries, and the left gastro-omental artery. Recall that the stomach and pancreas are foregut derivatives.

10. **C** The gallbladder is derived from the foregut. The hepatic diverticulum from the foregut divides into two parts; the larger cranial part gives rise to the liver, and the caudal part gives rise to the gallbladder.

11. **E** The celiac trunk (artery) carries blood from the aorta to the foregut derivatives (inferior end of the esophagus, stomach, liver, part of the duodenum, gallbladder, and part of the

pancreas). The celiac artery also supplies the spleen, which develops from mesenchyme in the dorsal mesentery of the stomach.

12. **B**  An umbilical sinus represents a remnant of the distal part of the yolk stalk at the umbilicus. A remnant of the proximal part of the yolk stalk is much more common and gives rise to an ileal (Meckel) diverticulum. Umbilical sinuses are lined by intestinal mucosa and secrete a mucoid material. They may be attached to the ileum by a fibrous cord (a remnant of the proximal part of the yolk stalk).

13. **B**  The duodenum is derived from the caudal part of the foregut and the cranial part of the midgut. The junction of the foregut and midgut is at the apex of the embryonic duodenal loop. The junction is indicated in the adult by the point of entrance of the bile duct. Because of its dual origin, the duodenum is supplied by both the foregut (celiac) and midgut (superior mesenteric) arteries.

14. **A**  The ventral mesentery between the cranial or superior part of the duodenum and the liver persists and gives rise to the hepatoduodenal ligament. The remainder of the ventral mesentery of the foregut gives rise to the hepatogastric ligament, peritoneal covering of the liver, falciform ligament, and coronary and triangular ligaments of the liver. The superior part of the duodenum is the only part of the intestines that has a ventral mesentery.

15. **D**  The liver arises as a diverticulum from the caudal end of the foregut. The proliferating endodermal cells give rise to interlacing cords of cells, which become the liver parenchyma. The fibrous and hematopoietic tissue are derived from splanchnic mesenchyme.

16. **C**  The visceral peritoneum of the liver is continuous with the hepatoduodenal ligament. This peritoneum is also continuous with the hepatogastric and falciform ligaments.

17. **E**  The umbilical vein passes in the inferior free border of the falciform ligament on its way to the liver with well-oxygenated blood from the placenta. Within the liver, the umbilical vein is broken up by the proliferating hepatic cords. The hepatic sinusoids are derived from remnants of the umbilical and vitelline veins. The adult derivative of the extrahepatic part of the umbilical vein is the round ligament (L. ligamentum teres) of the liver.

18. **D**  The liver is an important site of blood formation in the embryo and early fetus. Hematopoiesis begins in the liver during the sixth week; before this, blood formation occurs in the extraembryonic mesenchyme of the yolk sac and allantois. Blood is later formed in the spleen, bone marrow, and lymph nodes.

19. **C**  Esophageal atresia may occur as an isolated anomaly resulting from failure of canalization of the esophagus, but most often, it is associated with tracheoesophageal fistula. In more than 85% of cases of this type of fistula, the esophagus ends blindly. The fistula between the inferior end of the esophagus and the trachea results from faulty or incomplete partitioning of the foregut into the esophagus and the laryngotracheal tube. Incomplete formation of the tracheoesophageal septum at any level may give rise to a fistula.

20. **D**  Omphalocele is a congenital protrusion or herniation of the intestines through a large defect in the anterior abdominal wall at the umbilicus. This anomaly is believed to result from failure of the intestines to return from the umbilical cord during the tenth week. The hernial mass is covered by a thin, transparent membrane composed of peritoneum internally and amnion externally (from the amniotic covering of the umbilical cord).

21. **A**  Pyloric stenosis (narrowing of the distal opening of the stomach) results from hypertrophy of the muscle fibers of the pylorus, principally the circular musculature. The typical clinical picture is an infant who appears normal at birth, but within a week or more, there is a gradual onset of vomiting that progresses to a projectile type.

22. **E**  High intestinal obstruction (e.g., duodenal atresia) frequently is an accompaniment of polyhydramnios. Excessive amniotic fluid is

also associated with meroanencephaly (partial absence of the brain) and esophageal atresia. With meroanencephaly, there appears to be difficulty in swallowing. In esophageal and duodenal atresia, amniotic fluid accumulates because it is unable to pass to the intestines for absorption.

23. **A** Pyloric stenosis is the most common of all the anomalies listed. It affects male infants much more often than female infants. An incidence of 1:500 births represents an approximate overall average. It affects 1:150 males.

24. **B** Fistulas are associated with most cases of anorectal agenesis. The fistulas usually are rectourethral in males and rectovaginal in females. Anorectal agenesis with a fistula results from faulty or incomplete partitioning of the cloaca by the urorectal septum into the rectum and urogenital sinus.

# Urogenital System  13

## Objectives

Be able to:

- Discuss the development of the three sets of excretory organs, with emphasis on the permanent kidneys.
- Construct and label diagrams illustrating positional changes of the kidneys during development, briefly describing congenital anomalies of position and the renal vessels.
- Explain, with the aid of diagrams, the formation of the urinary bladder and urethra in both sexes.
- Describe the embryological basis of duplications of the superior part of the urinary tract, ectopic ureteral orifices, renal ectopia, horseshoe kidneys, congenital polycystic disease of the kidney, urachal anomalies, and exstrophy of the urinary bladder.
- Explain sex determination in human embryos and the meaning of the terms chromosomal sex, genetic sex, and phenotypic sex.
- Construct and label diagrams showing the development of the ovaries and testes, the genital ducts, and the external genitalia.
- Discuss the embryological basis of hypospadias and ambiguous external genitalia.
- Write brief notes on the appearance, migration, and significance of primordial germ cells; the development of the seminal and prostate glands; and clinically significant vestigial structures derived from the genital ducts.
- Discuss the embryological basis of intersexuality, and explain the terms true hermaphroditism and pseudohermaphroditism.
- Describe development of the suprarenal glands, and discuss congenital adrenocortical hyperplasia and its effects on the development of the external genitalia.
- Construct and label diagrams showing the development of the inguinal canals and descent of the testes.
- Explain the embryological basis of hydrocele and congenital inguinal hernia.

## Five-Choice Completion Questions

**Directions:** Each of the following statements or questions is followed by five suggested responses or completions. **Select the one best answer** in each case.

1. The human pronephros, a transitory nonfunctional "kidney," appears early in the fourth week as a few cell clusters in the _____ region of the embryo.

    A. occipital                      D. abdominal
    B. cervical                      E. pelvic
    C. thoracic

2. The human mesonephros, a transitory functional kidney, has largely degenerated by the _____ week.
   A. fifth
   B. sixth
   C. seventh
   D. eighth
   E. ninth

3. The metanephric diverticulum appears as a dorsal outgrowth from the
   A. mesonephric duct
   B. intermediate mesoderm
   C. urogenital sinus
   D. metanephric mesoderm
   E. cloaca

4. As the metanephric diverticulum grows dorsocranially, it is covered by _____ mesoderm
   A. splanchnic
   B. mesonephrogenic
   C. somatic
   D. metanephric
   E. intermediate

5. Incomplete division of the metanephric diverticulum before the renal pelvis forms results in
   A. bifid ureter
   B. supernumerary kidney
   C. duplication of the ureter
   D. partial ureteral duplication
   E. bifid ureter and supernumerary kidney

6. Embryologically, each uriniferous tubule consists of two parts, which become confluent at the junction of the
   A. renal corpuscle and the proximal convoluted tubule
   B. proximal convoluted tubule and the nephron loop
   C. descending and ascending limbs of the nephron loop
   D. ascending limb of the nephron loop and the distal convoluted tubule
   E. distal convoluted tubule and the collecting tubule

7. Exstrophy of the bladder often is associated with
   A. adrenal hyperplasia
   B. urachal fistula
   C. hypospadias
   D. epispadias
   E. chromosomal abnormalities

8. The metanephric diverticulum is derived from the
   A. urogenital sinus
   B. splanchnic mesoderm
   C. metanephric mesoderm
   D. somatic mesoderm
   E. mesonephric duct

9. Variations of the renal arteries are relatively common, and accessory vessels may compress the ureter, resulting in hydronephrosis and other complications. Supernumerary renal arteries are
   A. incompatible with postnatal life
   B. formed during the "descent" of the kidneys from the abdomen to the pelvis
   C. branches of the suprarenal arteries
   D. terminal or end arteries
   E. the cause of abnormal rotation of the kidneys

10. Unilateral renal agenesis was detected by ultrasonography in a near-term fetus that was associated with oligohydramnios. Failure of the kidney to develop probably resulted from
    A. unilateral polycystic disease
    B. degeneration of the mesonephros
    C. ureteric duplication
    D. failure of a metanephric diverticulum to form
    E. oligohydramnios

11. A male infant with hypospadias was referred to the urologist. This developmental anomaly
    A. results from defective formation of the genital tubercle
    B. is associated with exstrophy of the bladder
    C. involves the scrotum in most cases
    D. results from inadequate androgen production by the fetal testes or lack of adequate receptor sites for the hormones
    E. occurs in about 1:3000 male infants

12. Primordial germ cells are first recognizable early in the fourth week in the
    A. dorsal mesentery
    B. primary sex cords
    C. wall of the yolk sac
    D. gonadal ridges
    E. allantois

13. Cells of the cortical cords derived from the coelomic epithelium differentiate into
    A. follicular cells
    B. stromal cells
    C. oogonia
    D. theca folliculi
    E. primordial germ cells

14. The paramesonephric ducts in female embryos give rise to the
    A. paroöphoron
    B. uterine tubes
    C. inferior part of vagina
    D. round ligament of uterus
    E. ovarian ligament

15. The mesonephric duct in male embryos gives rise to the
    A. duct of epoöphoron
    B. duct of Gartner
    C. efferent ductule
    D. ductus deferens
    E. rete testis

16. The most common cause of female pseudohermaphroditism is
    A. maternal hormone ingestion
    B. adrenocortical hyperplasia
    C. maternal arrhenoblastoma
    D. maternal progestins
    E. testicular feminization

17. Which of the following cells are derived from mesenchyme?
    A. oogonia
    B. interstitial cells
    C. Sertoli cells
    D. follicular cells
    E. spermatogonia

18. Which of the following folds give rise to labia minora?
    A. genital
    B. labioscrotal
    C. urogenital
    D. urorectal
    E. labial

19. You are consulted about a neonate who was found to have chromatin-positive nuclei, ambiguous external genitalia, and an elevated 17-ketosteroid output. The most likely diagnosis is
    A. gonadal dysgenesis with chromosomal abnormalities
    B. female pseudohermaphroditism caused by maternal androgens
    C. male infant with perineal hypospadias
    D. congenital adrenocortical hyperplasia
    E. familial male pseudohermaphroditism

20. A neonate with an apparent perineal hypospadias was found to have chromatin-negative nuclei. Gonads were palpable in the inguinal canals. The mother previously had given birth to an apparent female child with ambiguous external genitalia. This girl, now 12 years old, shows strong signs of virilization. The most likely diagnosis of the condition in the present infant is
    A. female pseudohermaphroditism
    B. perineal hypospadias
    C. male pseudohermaphroditism
    D. gonadal dysgenesis
    E. true hermaphroditism

21. The urethral groove in the female fetus usually becomes the
    A. urethral orifice
    B. urethra
    C. navicular fossa
    D. frenulum of clitoris
    E. vestibule of vulva

22. A 14-year-old girl was admitted because of bilateral inguinal masses. She had not begun to menstruate but showed normal breast development for her age. Her external genitalia were feminine, the vagina was shallow, but no uterus could be palpated. Her sex chromatin pattern was negative. The most likely diagnosis is
    A. male pseudohermaphroditism
    B. female pseudohermaphroditism
    C. androgen insensitivity syndrome
    D. inguinal hernias
    E. Turner syndrome

23. A 16-year-old girl with a history of primary amenorrhea and cyclic pelvic pain was referred to a gynecologist. Careful examination revealed the presence of an imperforate hymen. This condition results from
    A. failure of the vaginal plate to canalize
    B. cervical atresia
    C. processus vaginalis
    D. androgen insensitivity syndrome
    E. failure of the sinovaginal bulbs to develop

24. A Gartner duct cyst was diagnosed in a female patient on routine pelvic examination. This condition develops from
    A. mesonephric duct
    B. mesonephric tubules
    C. paramesonephric duct
    D. urogenital folds
    E. none of the above

25. The feminization of the external genitalia is determined by the
    A. sinovaginal bulbs
    B. H-Y antigen
    C. ovaries
    D. absence of androgens
    E. epoöphoron

26. A bicornuate uterus was diagnosed in a 20-year-old patient who had been referred to a gynecologist because of several miscarriages. This uterine anomaly results from
    A. failure of fusion of the mesonephric ducts
    B. failure of the sinovaginal bulbs to fuse
    C. failure of fusion of the paramesonephric ducts
    D. absence of the urogenital sinus
    E. inadequate female hormones

27. A patient was diagnosed as having a supernumerary ovary. This condition is due to
    A. absence of the paramesonephric ducts
    B. delayed migration of the primordial germ cells
    C. the testis-determining factor
    D. the H-Y antigen
    E. absence of secondary sex cords

28. The interstitial cells (of Leydig)
    A. are derived from the surface epithelium
    B. secrete müllerian-inhibiting factor
    C. influence the differentiation of the ovary
    D. produce testosterone
    E. secrete progesterone

29. An imperforate hymen was diagnosed in an infant. This structure
    A. is a mucous membrane at the entrance to the vestibule of the vulva
    B. ruptures during the embryonic period
    C. separates the lumen of the vagina from the urogenital sinus in the fetus
    D. develops from the labia minora
    E. is formed by the paroöphoron

30. A mother brought her 6-month-old son to the doctor because the left testis was not in the scrotum. Formation of the testis is determined by
    A. SRY gene
    B. steroid hormones
    C. X chromosome inactivation
    D. retinoic acid
    E. *T-box* genes

## Answers and Explanations

1. **B**  The rudimentary pronephric "kidneys" appear in the cervical region. They have pronephric ducts that run caudally and open into the cloaca. The caudal parts of these ducts persist as the mesonephric ducts of the next set of kidneys that develop (the mesonephroi). In lower vertebrates, the pronephric ducts play an essential part in the induction of mesonephric tubules. They probably exert a similar influence in human embryos.

2. **E**  The mesonephros reaches its maximum development during the embryonic period. By the beginning of the fetal period (ninth week), most of the mesonephros has degenerated, except for its duct and a few tubules, which persist as genital ducts in males or rudimentary structures in females. By the time the mesonephroi have degenerated, the metanephroi or permanent kidneys have formed and have begun to function.

3. **A**  The metanephric diverticulum (ureteric bud) develops as a dorsal outgrowth from the mesonephric duct near its entry into the cloaca. The pronephric duct, which becomes the mesonephric duct, originally developed as an outgrowth from the intermediate mesoderm.

4. **D**  The metanephric mass of mesoderm, derived from the nephrogenic cord, forms a metanephrogenic cap over the expanded end or ampulla of the metanephric diverticulum. This mesenchyme gives rise to the nephrons. Differentiation of the nephrons is induced by an inductor substance produced by the ampulla of the ureteric bud and, later, the collecting tubules.

5. **C**  Incomplete division of the metanephric diverticulum (i.e., before the renal pelvis forms) usually results in the development of two ureters. One of the ureters may have an ectopic orifice; that is, it may open into the urethra in males or the vagina in females. Complete division of the metanephric diverticulum (before the calices form) results in incomplete ureteral duplication (i.e., bifid or **Y**-shaped ureter or double renal pelvis).

6. **E**  The nephron, consisting of a renal corpuscle and its associated tubules, develops from the metanephric mass of mesoderm around the collecting tubules. The end of a distal convoluted tubule of the nephron contacts and soon becomes confluent with a collecting tubule to form a uriniferous tubule.

7. **D**   Exstrophy of the urinary bladder often is associated with epispadias, a condition in which the urethra opens on the dorsal surface of the penis. This severe anomaly is very rare. In females with epispadias, there is a fissure in the urethra that opens on the dorsal surface of the clitoris.

8. **E**   The metanephric diverticulum develops as a hollow outgrowth from the mesonephric duct near its junction with the urogenital sinus. Shortly after it forms, the distal end of this outgrowth expands and comes into contact with the metanephric mesoderm of the most caudal part of the nephrogenic cord.

9. **D**   Supernumerary renal arteries are terminal or end arteries. If such an artery is damaged or ligated, the part of the kidney supplied by it becomes ischemic. As the kidney "ascends" from the pelvis into the abdomen, it continually acquires new branches from the aorta. Variations of the renal arteries reflect the persistence of these vessels, which normally disappear. Supernumerary renal arteries are compatible with postnatal life and play no part in the rotation of the kidneys.

10. **D**   Unilateral renal agenesis arises when the metanephric diverticulum on the ipsilateral side either is not formed or degenerates early. As a result, no nephrons are induced to form from the metanephric mesoderm. Whereas unilateral renal agenesis is relatively common and asymptomatic, bilateral renal agenesis is rare and fatal. The infant either is stillborn or dies almost immediately after birth.

11. **D**   Hypospadias is the most common abnormality of the male external genitalia. It occurs in about 1:300 male infants. Hypospadias results from incomplete fusion of the urogenital folds to form the spongy (penile) urethra. This is due to inadequate production of androgens by the fetal testes and/or insufficient receptor sites for the hormones. In most cases of hypospadias, the urethral orifice is on the ventral surface of the glans penis or on the ventral surface of the body of the penis. The scrotum is rarely involved. In severe forms of hypospadias, the penis usually is underdeveloped and curved ventrally, a condition known as chordee. Exstrophy of the bladder often is associated with epispadias, a less common defect in which the urethra opens on the dorsal surface of the penis.

12. **C**   The primordial germ cells are visible early in the fourth week between the endoderm and the mesoderm of the yolk sac, near the origin of the allantois. Later during the fourth week, as the yolk sac is partially incorporated into the embryo, the primordial germ cells migrate along the dorsal mesentery of the hindgut and enter the developing gonads. They give rise to the oogonia and spermatogonia in the ovaries and testes, respectively.

13. **A**   Cells of the coelomic epithelium give rise to cortical cords in female embryos that surround the primordial germ cells as they come from the yolk sac. The primordial germ cells become oogonia, and the coelomic epithelial cells become the follicular cells that surround the oogonia.

14. **B**   The paramesonephric ducts give rise to the uterine tubes and uterus. Some authors state that the superior four-fifths of the vagina is also formed from the paramesonephric ducts, but the majority opinion is that the vagina is derived from the urogenital sinus and the adjacent mesenchyme.

15. **D**   The mesonephric ducts give rise to the epididymis, ductus deferens, ejaculatory duct, and seminal glands.

16. **B**   The usual congenital form of the adrenogenital syndrome results from an inborn error of metabolism. The pituitary gland secretes excess corticotropin, causing hyperplasia of the fetal cortices of the suprarenal glands and an overproduction of androgens. These hormones cause masculinization of female fetuses (female pseudohermaphroditism). Masculinization of fetuses by hormones administered to pregnant females or produced by maternal adrenal tumors are uncommon causes of female pseudohermaphroditism.

17. **B**   The interstitial cells (of Leydig) develop from mesenchymal cells located between the developing seminiferous tubules. Some cells of this embryonic connective tissue enlarge and

group together to form clusters of interstitial cells. These cells produce androgens during fetal life that masculinize the genital ducts and external genitalia of males. The oogonia and spermatogonia develop from primordial germ cells; the follicular and Sertoli cells develop from the primary sex cords derived from the coelomic epithelium.

18. **C** The urogenital folds in the female fetus usually do not fuse but develop into the labia minora. In the presence of androgenic substances, they may fuse. In males, the urogenital folds fuse, closing the urethral groove and forming the spongy urethra.

19. **D** An elevated 17-ketosteroid output in a chromosomal female infant with ambiguous genitalia strongly indicates congenital adrenocortical hyperplasia. These infants have an enlarged clitoris, fused labia majora, and a persistent urogenital sinus. The virilization results from an excessive production of androgens by the hyperplastic suprarenal glands.

20. **C** In the case presented, the apparent female infant was a male pseudohermaphrodite. Were it not for the family history of intersexuality, the most likely diagnosis would be hypospadias. The cause of this condition is either a deficiency in the production of androgens or a defect in end-organ responsiveness to androgens.

21. **E** The urogenital folds usually do not fuse in females, and the urethral groove between them persists as the vestibule of the vulva (the space between the labia minora). The urethra and vagina open into the vestibule.

22. **C** The androgen insensitivity syndrome (formerly called the testicular feminization syndrome) often is considered a form of male pseudohermaphroditism, but these females do not have ambiguous external genitalia; hence, **C** is the best answer. The condition is uncommon and determined by a recessive gene. This kind of female would not pass the sex test given to females who register for the Olympics because of her chromatin-negative cells and male sex chromosome complement. In view of her female appearance and body structure, this is unjust.

23. **A** The vaginal plate — formed from the sinovaginal bulbs — gives rise to the vagina and the hymen. Imperforate hymen results from a failure of the inferior end of the vaginal plate to canalize. An imperforate hymen leads to hematocolpos, the accumulation of blood produced each month by the cyclic changes of a functional endometrium. The hymen usually presents itself on examination as a bulging, bluish membrane at the entrance to the vagina.

24. **A** Gartner duct cyst is formed from a remnant at the caudal end of the mesonephric duct. It is usually asymptomatic and is found in the wall of the vagina. The mesonephric tubules regress in the female, leaving some rudimentary tubules, the epoöphoron and paroöphoron. The uterine tubes, uterus, and vagina are derived from the paramesonephric ducts. The labia minora develop from the urogenital folds.

25. **D** The sinovaginal bulbs give rise to the vagina. The H-Y antigen directs the formation of seminiferous tubules from the primary sex cords; its absence in the female embryo results in the development of the ovaries. Sexual differentiation of the female external genitalia results from a lack of androgens or from androgen insensitivity. The epoöphoron is a mesonephric remnant in females.

26. **C** The uterus develops from the fusion of the paired paramesonephric ducts, followed by degeneration of the intervening septum. Duplication of the uterus results from a failure of this process, and it may result in two separate uteri. The mesonephric duct does not contribute to the development of the female genital tract, except for some vestigial remnants. The sinovaginal bulbs fuse and form the vaginal plate. The urinary bladder, urethra, vagina, urethral and paraurethral glands, as well as the greater vestibular glands, are derived from the urogenital sinus.

27. **B** A supernumerary ovary is an extremely rare gynecologic condition. About 20 cases have been reported in the medical literature. It results from an arrest in the migration of primordial germ cells along the dorsal mesentery of the hindgut to the genital ridges. An ectopic ovary may develop from these primordial germ

cells and the surrounding mesenchyme. The paramesonephric ducts give rise to the female genital tract. The testis-determining factor influences gonadal sex differentiation; and the H-Y antigen is involved in the formation of seminiferous tubules from the primary sex cords.

28. **D** The interstitial cells (of Leydig) are derived from mesenchymal cells. By the eighth week, these cells begin to produce the androgenic hormone testosterone, which is responsible for the differentiation of the male genital ducts and external genitalia. Progesterone is secreted by the corpus luteum. Müllerian-inhibiting factor, which is produced by the sustentacular cells (of Sertoli), suppresses the development of the paramesonephric duct in the male. The development of the ovary is not influenced by the interstitial cells.

29. **C** The hymen is a thin fold of mucous membrane at the entrance to the vagina. It usually ruptures during the perinatal period. A condition known as imperforate hymen results when this fails to occur. The incidence of imperforate hymen is about 0.1% or less. Fluid accumulation (hydrocolpos and hydrometrocolpos), especially at menarche, leads to a characteristic protruding of the membrane at the entrance to the vagina. The paroöphoron is not involved in the formation of the hymen. It is a mesonephric remnant in females.

30. **A** The SRY gene (testis determining factor) in the short arm of the Y chromosome initiates testicular development in the gonadal ridge of the embryo. SRY encodes a zinc-finger transcription factor which regulates the expression of other genes.

# Five-Choice Association Questions

**Directions:** Each group of questions below consists of a numbered list of descriptive words or phrases accompanied by a diagram with certain parts indicated by letters or by a list of lettered headings. For each numbered word or phrase, **select the lettered part or heading** that matches it correctly and then insert the letter in the space to the right of the appropriate number. Sometimes more than one numbered word or phrase may be correctly matched to the same lettered part or heading.

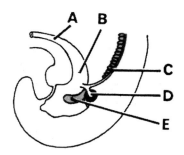

A. Renal agenesis
B. Nephrogenic cord
C. Metanephric diverticulum
D. Kidney lobes
E. Polycystic kidney

1. _____ Urogenital sinus
2. _____ Gives rise to collecting system of kidney
3. _____ Partitions the cloaca
4. _____ Primordium of renal pelvis and calices
5. _____ Becomes median umbilical ligament
6. _____ Degenerates in females
7. _____ Vestigial structure in human embryos
8. _____ Temporary embryonic kidney

9. _____ Source of nephrons
10. _____ Caused by dilations of the nephron loops
11. _____ Oligohydramnios
12. _____ Mesonephric duct
13. _____ Intermediate mesoderm
14. _____ External evidence of them disappears during infancy

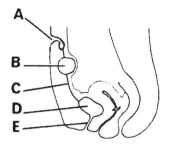

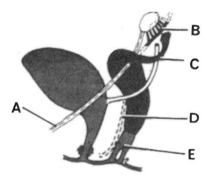

A. Adrenal hyperplasia
B. Penile hypospadias
C. Zona reticularis
D. Neuroectoderm
E. Coelomic epithelium

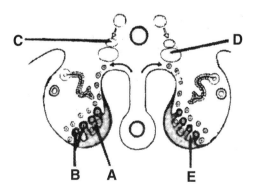

A. Urogenital folds
B. Rete testis
C. Glandular plate
D. Genital tubercle
E. External oblique aponeurosis

15. _____ Opens at the umbilicus
16. _____ May undergo exstrophy
17. _____ Becomes the median umbilical ligament
18. _____ Urachal sinus
19. _____ Cystic remnant of the urachus
20. _____ Short tube derived from urogenital sinus and splanchnic mesenchyme

21. _____ Derivative of paramesonephric duct
22. _____ Corresponds to the epididymis
23. _____ Passes through the inguinal canal
24. _____ Composed of endodermal cells
25. _____ Derivative of the gubernaculum
26. _____ Derivative of the urogenital sinus
27. _____ Epoöphoron
28. _____ Gartner duct cyst

29. _____ Suprarenal medulla
30. _____ Gives rise to suprarenal cortex
31. _____ Differentiates after birth
32. _____ Unfused urogenital folds
33. _____ Ambiguous external genitalia
34. _____ Associated with chordee

35. _____ Primordium of suprarenal medulla
36. _____ Gives rise to interstitial cells
37. _____ Primary sex cord
38. _____ Primordium of suprarenal cortex
39. _____ Give rise to oogonia
40. _____ Degenerates in females

41. _____ External spermatic fascia
42. _____ Gives rise to the clitoris
43. _____ Primary sex cords in males
44. _____ Hypospadias
45. _____ Navicular fossa
46. _____ Labia minora

## Answers and Explanations

1. **B** The urogenital sinus gives rise to the epithelium of the urinary bladder. Distally, it also gives rise to the epithelium of the urethra, except for the terminal part of the spongy urethra (navicular fossa); this part is derived from surface ectoderm. Other parts of the walls of these structures differentiate from the adjacent splanchnic mesenchyme.

2. **D** The metanephric diverticulum gives rise to the collecting system of the kidney (i.e., the ureter, renal pelvis, calices, and collecting tubules). As the diverticulum grows dorsocranially, it slowly invades the metanephric mass of mesoderm. This mesenchyme stimulates the metanephric diverticulum to differentiate into calices and other parts of the collecting system of the permanent kidney. These structures then induce the mesenchyme to differentiate into nephrons.

3. **E** The urorectal septum is a coronal wedge of mesenchyme between the allantois and the hindgut. As it grows toward the cloacal membrane, it produces infoldings of the lateral walls of the cloaca. When these infoldings fuse, they divide the cloaca into the rectum dorsally and the urogenital sinus ventrally. The urorectal septum also divides the cloacal membrane into the anal membrane and the urogenital membrane. The area of fusion of the urorectal septum with the cloacal membrane becomes the perineal body (tendinous center of perineum).

4. **D** The metanephric diverticulum is the primordium of the renal pelvis, calices, and collecting tubules. The metanephric mesenchyme stimulates the ampulla (future renal pelvis) of the diverticulum to divide into the calices and the collecting tubules to grow into the metanephric mesenchyme from the cuplike calices. Subsequently, these tubules contact and become confluent with the nephrons to form uriniferous tubules.

5. **A** The allantois becomes the urachus in the fetus and forms the median umbilical ligament in the adult. Remnants of the allantois that do not become ligamentous may give rise to urachal sinuses, fistulas, or cysts. Urachal remnants are not usually detected unless they become infected.

6. **C** The mesonephros degenerates in females; almost all of it also degenerates in males. Some caudal mesonephric tubules persist in males as the efferent ductules of the testis. Before the mesonephros degenerates, the metanephric diverticulum grows from the mesonephric duct and forms the collecting system of the kidneys. Remnants of mesonephric tubules and the mesonephric duct may persist in females and give rise to cysts (e.g., cysts of the epoöphoron).

7. **A** The allantois is a vestigial structure in the human embryo; it develops during the second week as a diverticulum from the caudal wall of the yolk sac. In some species it serves as a reservoir for excretory products, but in the human embryo it remains small and becomes the urachus in the fetus and the median umbilical ligament in the adult. Although it may contribute to the apex of the urinary bladder, it is believed that the entire bladder develops from the urogenital sinus and the adjacent mesenchyme.

8. **C** The mesonephros is the second kidney to develop in the human embryo. The first one (pronephros) is rudimentary, but the mesonephros is believed to function for a few weeks while the metanephros or permanent kidney is developing.

9. **B** The metanephric mesenchyme in the nephrogenic cords gives rise to nephrons. When stimulated by a substance produced by the metanephric diverticulum, the metanephric mesenchyme begins to differentiate into nephrons.

10. **E** Congenital polycystic disease of the kidneys is transmitted on an autosomal basis (ARPKD). The cysts may result from failure of the first formed rudimentary nephrons to degenerate; later, these remnants may accumulate fluid and form cysts. Cysts may also develop from detached parts of metanephric tissue, which gives rise to rudimentary renal vesicles. It is now widely believed that these cysts are dilations of the nephrons, particularly of the nephron loops.

11. **A** Oligohydramnios (an abnormally small volume of amniotic fluid) may be associated with renal agenesis (absence of kidneys). In the neonate, renal agenesis is suggested by large, low-set ears. This type of auricle also suggests numerical chromosomal abnormalities (e.g., trisomy 18). The fetal kidneys normally

produce large amounts of urine, which is excreted into the amniotic fluid. When one or both kidneys fail to form or there is urethral obstruction, the volume of amniotic fluid is small because urine production fails to occur or the urine cannot pass into the amniotic fluid.

12. **C** The metanephric diverticulum develops as an outgrowth of the mesonephric duct near its opening into the urogenital sinus. This diverticulum gives rise to the ureter, renal pelvis, calices, and collecting tubules.

13. **B** The intermediate mesoderm in the early embryo forms a longitudinal mass on each side called the nephrogenic cord. These cords give rise to nephrons, which connect with the collecting tubules formed from the metanephric diverticula.

14. **D** The external evidence of the kidney lobes disappears during infancy, usually by the end of the first year. Thereafter, lobes are observed only in sections of the kidney and are defined as a medullary pyramid with its cap of cortical tissue.

15. **A** A urachal sinus may open at the umbilicus and produce a discharge. The allantois, running between the umbilicus and the urinary bladder, usually becomes the urachus and, eventually, the median umbilical ligament. If the cranial part of the allantois remains patent, a sinus may form. More often, the caudal end of the allantois remains patent and gives rise to a sinus that may be continuous with the cavity of the urinary bladder.

16. **D** The posterior wall of the urinary bladder may protrude through a defect in the anterior abdominal wall; this defect is called exstrophy of the bladder. The trigone and ureteral orifices are exposed, and urine dribbles intermittently.

17. **C** The urachus, a derivative of the allantois, usually becomes a fibrous cord after birth — the median umbilical ligament, which extends from the apex of the urinary bladder to the umbilicus.

18. **A** Failure of closure of a part of the intra-embryonic part of the allantois may result in the formation of a urachal sinus that opens at the umbilicus or into the urinary bladder. These sinuses usually are not detected unless they become infected and produce a discharge at the umbilicus or a bladder infection.

19. **B** Remnants of the urachus that do not become fibrous and form the median umbilical ligament may accumulate fluid and become cystic. Small cysts commonly are detected in sections of the urachus or median umbilical ligament, but most cysts are not detected in living people unless they become infected and enlarge.

20. **E** The urethra in the female is a short tube that extends from the urinary bladder to the external orifice. The epithelium of the urethra is derived from the endodermal urogenital sinus; all other layers of its wall are derived from the adjacent splanchnic mesenchyme.

21. **C** The uterine tube is a derivative of the para-mesonephric duct. The fused parts of these ducts give rise to the uterus.

22. **B** The epoöphoron appears in the broad ligament between the ovary and the uterine tube. It is a remnant of the mesonephric duct and some mesonephric tubules and is homologous with the epididymis in males. It may become cystic and give rise to a large parovarian cyst.

23. **A** The round ligament of the uterus passes through the inguinal canal and attaches to the labium majus. It is continuous with the ovarian ligament because they are both derived from the embryonic gubernaculum.

24. **E** The vaginal plate is composed of endodermal cells derived from the urogenital sinus. Later, the central cells of this plate break down, forming the lumen of the vagina. Failure of this canalization to occur results in vaginal atresia.

25. **A** The round ligament is a derivative of the gubernaculum, a fibromuscular cord that passes from the inferior pole of the gonad. It descends obliquely through the developing abdominal wall (future site of the inguinal canal) and attaches to the labioscrotal fold (future labium majus).

26. **E**   The vaginal plate is derived from a pair of sinovaginal bulbs that grow out from the urogenital sinus and fuse to form a solid cord of endodermal cells called the vaginal plate. The central cells of this plate subsequently degenerate, forming the lumen of the vagina.

27. **B**   The epoöphoron is a vestigial structure that lies in the broad ligament between the ovary and the uterine tube. It consists of a few blind tubules connected to a short duct. If the epoöphoron becomes distended with fluid, it forms a parovarian cyst. Most are small, but some are very large.

28. **D**   Gartner duct cysts are derived from remnants of caudal parts of the mesonephric duct in females. They are located between the layers of the broad ligament along the lateral wall of the uterus or in the wall of the vagina. Gartner duct cysts seldom are detected unless they become infected and enlarged.

29. **D**   The medulla of the suprarenal gland is derived from neuroectoderm. Neural crest cells, comparable to those that form sympathetic ganglia, invade the mesodermal suprarenal cortex on its medial side and soon become surrounded by it.

30. **E**   The fetal suprarenal cortex is derived from mesenchymal cells that arise from the coelomic epithelium. These large cells make up most of the suprarenal cortex before birth, forming the massive fetal cortex. The fetal cortex gradually involutes after birth and usually is not recognizable after the first year.

31. **C**   At birth, the suprarenal gland consists mainly of fetal cortex. The zona reticularis of the adrenal cortex forms after birth. It usually is recognizable by the end of the third year. The other two layers of the permanent cortex (zona glomerulosa and zona fasciculata) are present at birth but are not fully differentiated.

32. **B**   Failure of the urogenital folds to fuse in males results in hypospadias. In most cases, the urethra opens on the ventral surface near the junction of the glans and the body of the penis.

33. **A**   Ambiguous external genitalia often indicate virilization of a female, resulting from congenital virilizing adrenal hyperplasia. Excessive production of adrenal androgens by the hyperplastic fetal cortices of the suprarenal glands causes masculinization of the external genitalia. A neonate with ambiguous genitalia, a palpable uterus, but no palpable gonads usually is a female pseudohermaphrodite whose condition is caused by adrenocortical hyperplasia.

34. **B**   Chordee, a curving downward of the penis, often is associated with hypospadias, especially with the more severe types (e.g., penoscrotal hypospadias).

35. **C**   The medulla of the suprarenal gland is derived from neuroectoderm. Neural crest cells, comparable to those that give rise to sympathetic nerve cells, migrate to the developing suprarenal cortex and later give rise to the suprarenal medulla.

36. **E**   The mesenchyme, separating the primary sex cords, gives rise to the interstitial cells. Some cells of the mesenchyme enlarge and become grouped together. They produce androgens during the fetal period that stimulate development of the mesonephric ducts and inhibit development of the paramesonephric ducts. These sex hormones also cause masculinization of the external genitalia.

37. **A**   The primary sex cords give rise to the seminiferous tubules, tubuli recti, and rete testis. They lose their connections with the surface epithelium as the tunica albuginea forms.

38. **D**   The suprarenal cortex, derived from mesoderm, is first recognizable as a mass of mesenchymal cells on each side between the root of the mesentery and the developing gonad. Before birth, most of the suprarenal cortex consists of fetal cortex. This zone rapidly involutes after birth, losing about half its mass in 2 weeks.

39. **B**   The primordial germ cells are the precursors of oogonia in female embryos and spermatogonia in male embryos. The primordial germ cells migrate from the yolk sac to the gonads

and soon become incorporated into the primary sex cords.

40. **A**  The primary sex cords normally degenerate in female embryos, but during the fetal period, secondary sex cords or cortical cords extend from the surface epithelium into the underlying mesenchyme. Primordial germ cells are incorporated into the cortical cords and give rise to the oogonia. The follicular cells that surround the oogonia are derived from the cortical cords.

41. **E**  The external spermatic fascia is an extension of the external oblique aponeurosis. As the testis and its associated structures descend, they become ensheathed by fascial extensions of the abdominal wall. These extensions are produced by the processus vaginalis as it projects through the abdominal wall along the path formed by the gubernaculum.

42. **D**  The genital tubercle elongates in both sexes to form the phallus. In females, growth of the phallus normally slows after the eighth week; it becomes the relatively small clitoris. In the presence of androgenic substances (e.g., administered to the mother or produced by hyperplastic fetal suprarenal glands), the clitoris elongates to form a penislike structure and the labia majora fuse.

43. **B**  The primary sex cords in male embryos condense and extend into the medulla of the developing testis. Here they branch, and their ends anastomose to form the rete testis.

44. **A**  Hypospadias is a common anomaly of the urethra (occurring in about 1:300 males) resulting from failure of fusion of the urogenital folds. In some cases, the labioscrotal folds also fail to fuse and result in severe forms of hypospadias (e.g., penoscrotal and perineal hypospadias). This arrest of development is the result of an inadequate production of androgens by the fetal testes.

45. **C**  The terminal part of the penile urethra, the navicular fossa, is derived from the glandular plate. This plate is formed by an ectodermal ingrowth into the glans penis from the surface epithelium. Subsequent splitting of this plate forms a groove on the ventral surface of the glans. Closure of the urethral groove moves the external urethral orifice to the tip of the glans penis and joins this part of the spongy urethra with that formed by fusion of the urogenital folds.

46. **A**  The labia minora develop from the urogenital folds. In male embryos that receive adequate amounts of androgenic hormones, the urogenital folds fuse to form the spongy urethra.

# Cardiovascular System

## Objectives

Be able to:

- Illustrate with simple, labeled sketches the events occuring between the third and sixth weeks that change the primordial heart into the adult heart.
- Explain partitioning of the primordial atrium and ventricle, discussing clinically significant atrial and ventricular septal defects.
- Construct and label diagrams illustrating the course of the fetal circulation and the changes that occur at birth and during the postnatal period.
- Summarize the major events in the transformation of the embryonic aortic arch system into the adult arterial pattern.
- Discuss the relatively common aortic arch anomalies (especially patent ductus arteriosus and coarctation of the aorta).
- Outline the embryological basis of the following congenital anomalies: double aortic arch, right aortic arch, and retroesophageal subclavian artery.

## Five-Choice Completion Questions

**Directions:** Each of the following statements or questions is followed by five suggested responses or completions. **Select the one best answer** in each case.

1. Incomplete fusion of the endocardial cushions usually is associated with which of the following types of atrial septal defect (ASD)?
   - A. secundum-type ASD
   - B. primum-type ASD
   - C. common atrium
   - D. probe patent ASD
   - E. sinus venosus-type ASD

2. The fetal left atrium is mainly derived from the
   - A. primordial pulmonary vein
   - B. right pulmonary vein
   - C. primordial atrium
   - D. sinus venarum
   - E. sinus venosus

3. Congenital heart disease is the most common cardiac condition in childhood and most frequently results from
   - A. maternal medications
   - B. mutant genes
   - C. rubella virus
   - D. fetal distress
   - E. multifactorial inheritance

4. The most common type of defect of the cardiac septa is
    A. secundum-type ASD
    B. muscular-type VSD
    C. primum-type ASD
    D. membranous-type VSD
    E. sinus venosus-type ASD

5. Closure of the foramen primum results from fusion of the
    A. septum primum and septum secundum
    B. septum secundum and septum spurium
    C. septum primum and endocardial cushions
    D. septum secundum and endocardial cushions
    E. septum primum and right sinuatrial valve

6. The fetal right atrium is mainly derived from the
    A. primordial pulmonary vein
    B. right pulmonary vein
    C. primordial atrium
    D. sinus venarum
    E. sinus venosus

7. The most common congenital defect of the heart and great vessels associated with the congenital rubella syndrome is
    A. coarctation of the aorta          D. ASD
    B. tetralogy of Fallot                E. VSD
    C. patent ductus arteriosus

8. The cardiovascular system reaches a functional state at the end of the _____ week.
    A. second          D. fifth
    B. third           E. sixth
    C. fourth

9. A female infant with congestive heart failure and continuous systolic and diastolic murmurs was diagnosed as having a patent ductus arteriosus. Which of the following statements is correct?
    A. The ductus arteriosus is a remnant of the left fourth aortic arch.
    B. The ductus arteriosus closes during fetal development.
    C. The ductus arteriosus shunts blood from the umbilical vein to the inferior vena cava.
    D. The ductus arteriosus closes just before birth.
    E. In the fetus, most of the blood from the pulmonary trunk flows into the aorta.

10. On routine examination of an infant who has failed to thrive and has low weight, a loud murmur was detected at the lower left sternal border. A diagnosis of VSD was made, and subsequently, the absence of the membranous part of the atrioventricular septum was confirmed by two-dimensional echocardiography. Membranous VSD
    A. is the result of failure of subendocardial tissue of endocardial cushions to fuse with the aorticopulmonary septum and the muscular part of the interventricular septum
    B. results from excessive resorption of myocardial tissue during the embryonic period
    C. causes shunting of blood from the right ventricle into the left ventricle
    D. is found only in association with an ASD
    E. is the less common type of VSD

11. Transposition of the great arteries was diagnosed in a male infant with obvious cyanosis and mild tachypnea. This condition results from
    A. abnormal resorption of the septum primum
    B. failure of the endocardial cushions to fuse
    C. faulty partitioning of the bulbus cordis and truncus arteriosus
    D. involution of the ductus arteriosus
    E. abnormal transformation of the sixth aortic arches

12. A secundum ASD was detected in a young child. This congenital defect
    A. occurs more frequently in males than in females
    B. is located near the superior vena cava
    C. results from abnormal resorption of the septum primum
    D. usually causes death in early childhood
    E. includes defects of the fused endocardial cushions

13. Dextrocardia was diagnosed in an infant. The signaling factor most likely to be involved in this defect is
    A. angiopoietin
    B. bone morphogenetic proteins
    C. retinoic acid
    D. engrailed 1 and 2
    E. nodal

## Answers and Explanations

1. **B** The primum-type ASD associated with an endocardial cushion defect is the second most common type of clinically significant ASD. The incomplete form of endocardial cushion defect is relatively common, in which the septum primum does not fuse with the endocardial cushions. As a result, there is a patent oval foramen and often a cleft in the anterior leaflet of the mitral valve.

2. **A** Most of the wall of the left atrium is smooth and derived by absorption of the primordial pulmonary vein. At first, the common pulmonary vein opens into the primordial left atrium, but as the atrium expands, parts of this vein are incorporated into the wall of the atrium. The primordial atrium forms only a relatively small part of the adult left atrium (i.e., the left auricle).

3. **E** Congenital heart disease usually is not caused by a single factor. Heart anomalies may result from single-gene disorders, but most fit the criteria for multifactorial inheritance. Rubella virus is known to be associated with patent ductus arteriosus and pulmonary stenosis. Maternal medications (e.g., thalidomide) rarely are associated with congenital heart disease; however, most heart defects result from unknown causes, probably a complex interaction of genetic and environmental factors.

4. **D** Membranous-type VSD is the most common type of heart defect. This anomaly usually results from failure of the membranous part of the interventricular septum to form at the end of the seventh week. The formation of this part of the septum results from fusion of tissues from three sources.

5. **C** As the septum primum grows toward the fusing endocardial cushions, the foramen primum becomes progressively smaller. The septum primum eventually fuses with the left side of the fused endocardial cushions and obliterates the foramen primum. This type of ASD is less common than a patent oval foramen.

6. **E**  Most of the wall of the right atrium is smooth and derived by absorption of the right horn of the sinus venosus. The sinus venosus initially opens into the right atrium but as the atrium expands, the right horn of the sinus venosus gradually is incorporated into the right atrium and becomes the smooth-walled part — the sinus venarum. The primordial atrium is represented by the right auricle, a small muscular pouch. The smooth part (sinus venarum) and the rough part (auricle) are demarcated internally by a vertical ridge, the crista terminalis or terminal crest, and externally by a shallow inconspicuous groove, the sulcus terminalis or terminal groove.

7. **C**  The most frequent anomalies associated with the congenital rubella syndrome are congenital heart defects (especially patent ductus arteriosus and pulmonary stenosis), deafness, and blindness (cataract). These anomalies result from maternal infection during the first trimester of pregnancy. Rubella infection during the second trimester can cause deafness, microcephaly, and mental retardation. The influence of teratogens such as rubella on development of the heart and great vessels is well known, but the role of other viral infections and drugs is inconclusive.

8. **B**  Cardiovascular development is first evident in the cardiogenic area at about 18 days. By the end of the third week, embryonic and extra-embryonic vessels are connected to the heart and a slow circulation of blood has begun. When the heart begins to beat about a day later, the circulation becomes an ebb and flow type.

9. **E**  The ductus arteriosus is derived from the left sixth aortic arch; the left fourth aortic arch contributes to the formation of the arch of the aorta. In the fetus, the lumen of the ductus arteriosus is large and permits the flow of blood from the pulmonary trunk into the aorta. Pulmonary blood flow in the fetus is low because of the high pulmonary resistance. The ductus arteriosus constricts at birth and usually is functionally closed 10 to 15 hours later. With involution, it becomes the ligamentum arteriosum. A patent ductus arteriosus (PDA) is more commonly found in females than in males. With only few exceptions, all patients with PDA require medical or surgical closure of the ductus.

10. **A**  VSD is the most common type of cardiac anomaly, and a defect in the membranous part of the septum is the most common type of VSD. It is caused by a failure of the subendocardial tissues of the fused endocardial cushions to fuse with both the aorticopulmonary septum and the muscular part of the interventricular septum. VSDs are embryologically unrelated to ASDs. A VSD causes shunting of left ventricular blood into the right ventricle. Spontaneous closure of VSDs during the first few months after birth is relatively common, but in other cases, medical management or surgery is indicated to deal with the accompanying congestive heart failure.

11. **C**  It is believed that failure of the aorticopulmonary septum to pursue a spiral course during the division of the bulbus cordis and the truncus arteriosus results in the aorta arising from the right ventricle and the pulmonary trunk from the left ventricle. This is one of the most common cardiac defects seen in infancy, predominantly in males. Other congenital cardiac defects may be present in neonates with transposition of the great vessels.

12. **C**  Secundum ASDs occur more frequently in females than in males (3:1). The lesions are located in the area of the oval fossa and involve both the septum primum and septum secundum. Children with ASDs are usually asymptomatic, and only later symptoms may appear. Abnormal resorption of the septum primum during formation of the septum secundum, excessive resorption of the septum primum, or defective development of the septum secundum provides an embryological explanation for secundum ASDs.

13. **E**  Nodal, a member of the FGF-β superfamily, is asymmetrically expressed in vertebrate mesoderm and plays an essential role in mesodermal patterning. Because nodal regulates looping of the heart tube, it has been suggested that disturbance in nodal expression might be involved in dextrocardia and situs inversus.

# *Five-Choice Association Questions*

**Directions:** Each group of questions below consists of a numbered list of descriptive words or phrases accompanied by a diagram with certain parts indicated by letters or by a list of lettered headings. For each numbered word or phrase, **select the lettered part or heading** that matches it correctly, and then insert the letter in the space to the right of the appropriate number. Sometimes more than one numbered word or phrase may be correctly matched to the same lettered part or heading.

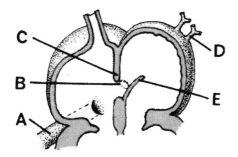

A. Ductus arteriosus
B. Septum primum
C. Sixth aortic arch
D. Sinus venosus
E. Umbilical vein

1. _____ Directs blood into the left atrium
2. _____ Carry relatively little fetal blood
3. _____ Remains of the septum primum
4. _____ Opening in the septum secundum
5. _____ Carries well-oxygenated blood
6. _____ Septum secundum

7. _____ Round ligament of liver
8. _____ Carries poorly oxygenated blood into the right atrium
9. _____ Arterial shunt
10. _____ Floor of the oval fossa
11. _____ Ductus venosus
12. _____ Right recurrent laryngeal nerve

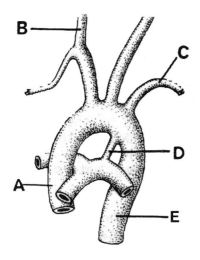

A. Coarctation
B. Infundibular stenosis
C. Patent ductus arteriosus
D. VSD
E. Tetralogy of Fallot

13. _____ Derivative of an intersegmental artery
14. _____ Forms from the sixth aortic arch artery
15. _____ Derived from the truncus arteriosus
16. _____ Formed by fusion of the dorsal aortae
17. _____ Derived from the third aortic arch artery
18. _____ Becomes ligamentous during infancy

19. _____ Pulmonary valve stenosis
20. _____ Rubella syndrome
21. _____ Right ventricular hypertrophy
22. _____ Most common cardiac defect
23. _____ Constriction of aorta
24. _____ Overriding aorta

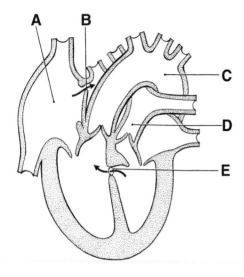

25. _____ A cardiac defect in the area of the oval fossa
26. _____ Normally communicates with the right ventricle
27. _____ Closes by the end of the seventh embryonic week
28. _____ Is formed from the dorsal aorta
29. _____ Is partly derived from the sinus venosus

---

## Answers and Explanations

1. **C**  Blood from the inferior vena cava (IVC) is directed by the inferior border of the septum secundum (crista dividens) through the oval foramen into the left atrium.

2. **D**  The pulmonary veins carry relatively little blood to the left atrium before birth because the lungs are not functioning. When the lungs expand at birth and the pulmonary vascular resistance falls, there is a marked increase in pulmonary blood flow with a consequent increased flow of oxygenated blood to the left atrium through the pulmonary veins.

3. **E**  The remains of the septum primum are represented in the drawing by the valve of the oval foramen. This valve is forced open by blood from the IVC that is directed through the oval foramen by the crista dividens (inferior edge of septum secundum). The oval foramen normally closes at birth when pressure in the left atrium rises above that in the right atrium.

4. **B**  The oval foramen is a normal opening in the septum secundum. It permits well-oxygenated blood from the placenta that comes from the IVC to enter the left atrium. If the oval foramen fails to close at birth, a cardiac anomaly known as secundum-type ASD exists. This common congenital heart defect accounts for about 8% of cases of congenital heart disease.

5. **A**  The IVC carries well-oxygenated blood from the placenta. This fetal blood returns from the placenta in the umbilical vein. About half the blood passes through the hepatic sinusoids before entering the IVC. The other half is shunted by way of the ductus venosus directly from the umbilical vein to the IVC.

6. **C**  The septum secundum is the second part of the interatrial septum to form. The crista dividens, its inferior border, is indicated by the pointer. It directs most of the blood from the IVC through the opening in the septum secundum (oval foramen) into the left atrium. The smaller portion of blood, turned back by the septum secundum, enters the right ventricle.

7. **E**  The intra-abdominal part of the fetal umbilical vein becomes the adult round ligament of the liver (L. ligamentum teres hepatis). It passes from the umbilicus to the porta hepatis, where it attaches to the left branch of the portal vein.

8. **D**  The sinus venosus initially is a separate chamber of the heart that opens into the caudal wall of the right atrium. The right horn of the sinus venosus becomes incorporated into the wall of the right atrium and forms its smooth-walled part called the sinus venarum. The left horn of the sinus venosus becomes the coronary sinus.

9. **A** The ductus arteriosus is an arterial shunt that carries blood from the left pulmonary artery to the arch of the aorta before birth. Because the lungs are not functioning, most of the blood in the pulmonary trunk bypasses the lungs and enters the descending aorta.

10. **B** The floor of the oval fossa in the interatrial septum is formed by tissue derived from the septum primum (valve of oval foramen). When the pressure in the left atrium rises at birth, the valve of the oval foramen closes and later fuses with the septum secundum. This valvular tissue forms the floor of the oval fossa.

11. **E** About half the blood coming from the placenta in the umbilical vein is shunted through the liver by way of the ductus venosus into the IVC. The remainder of the blood enters the liver and is carried to the IVC by the hepatic veins.

12. **C** The recurrent laryngeal nerves hook around the sixth pair of aortic arch arteries. On the right, the distal part of the sixth arch artery and the fifth aortic arch artery degenerate, leaving the right recurrent laryngeal nerve hooked around the right subclavian artery. On the left, the recurrent laryngeal nerve hooks around the ductus arteriosus (ligamentum arteriosum in the adult) and the arch of the aorta.

13. **C** The left subclavian artery, unlike the right subclavian artery, is not derived from an aortic arch artery or the dorsal aorta. It develops from the seventh intersegmental artery that arises from the descending aorta and moves cranially as the arch of the aorta forms.

14. **D** The ductus arteriosus develops from the distal portion of the left sixth aortic arch artery. It passes from the left pulmonary artery to the aorta and, before birth, carries most of the blood from the pulmonary trunk into the aorta. The lungs are not functioning and so require little blood. The ductus arteriosus usually constricts slightly after birth and closes anatomically during the first 3 months.

15. **A** The proximal part of the ascending aorta is derived from the truncus arteriosus when it is divided by the aorticopulmonary septum. The remainder of the ascending aorta develops from the aortic sac.

16. **E** The descending aorta forms when the paired dorsal aortae of the embryo fuse. The cranial part of the right dorsal aorta normally involutes, but if it persists, a double aortic arch forms that may compress the trachea and esophagus.

17. **B** The right common carotid artery is derived from the proximal part of the right third aortic arch artery. This artery also gives rise to the internal carotid artery on this side.

18. **D** The ductus arteriosus constricts at birth but usually is patent for a week or so. Proliferation of endothelial and fibrous tissues of the ductus arteriosus usually results in its anatomic closure by the end of the third month.

19. **E** Stenosis of the pulmonary tract is one of the four anomalies of the heart and great vessels included in the tetralogy of Fallot. These defects are regarded as the most important of the cardiac defects that produce cyanosis.

20. **C** Patent ductus arteriosus is the most common congenital anomaly of the heart and great vessels associated with maternal rubella infection during the first trimester.

21. **B** Enlargement and hypertrophy of the right ventricle result from high blood pressure, often resulting from pulmonary stenosis. The narrowing may occur at the infundibulum of the right ventricle, the pulmonary valve, or, less commonly, in the pulmonary trunk. **E** is also correct, but **B** is the better answer.

22. **D** VSD is the most common cardiac defect. It may occur with various other cardiac defects (e.g., in tetralogy of Fallot). VSD most commonly consists of an opening (1 to 15 mm in diameter) in the membranous part of the interventricular septum.

23. **A** In preductal coarctation, the aorta constricts superior to the ductus arteriosus, which usually is patent. More often, the constriction is inferior to the ductus (postductal coarctation).

24. **E** Overriding aorta or an aorta arising directly over a VSD, and thus overriding both ventricular cavities, is an essential feature of the tetralogy of Fallot. People with this group of cardiac defects are cyanotic because not enough blood flows to the lungs for oxygenation. As long as the ductus arteriosus remains patent, there is compensatory flow through it from the aorta to the pulmonary arteries. If the ductus closes, as commonly occurs, the deficit in pulmonary circulation increases.

25. **B** Atrial septal defect (ASD) is a common congenital anomaly. It occurs more frequently in females than in males. A patent oval foramen is the most common form of ASD, resulting from incomplete fusion between the septum secundum and the flap-type valve of the oval foramen. Before birth, most of the blood entering the right atrium is shunted through the oval foramen into the left atrium. After birth, the pressure in the left atrium rises with the return of blood from the lungs. As a result, the septum primum becomes pressed against the septum secundum, and eventually the oval foramen is permanently closed. Of the main types of ASD, the secundum ASD is most common and is located in the area of the oval fossa.

26. **D** The pulmonary trunk normally communicates with the right ventricle, transporting poorly oxygenated blood to the lungs after birth. In typical cases of transposition of the great arteries, the aorta arises from the right ventricle anteriorly, and on the left the pulmonary artery arises from the left ventricle posteriorly. Transposition of the great arteries is the most common cause of cyanotic heart disease in newborn infants, and it is often found in association with other cardiac anomalies.

27. **E** A crescentic interventricular foramen, between the free edge of the muscular part of the interventricular septum and the fused endocardial cushions, permits blood to pass between the right and left ventricles until the seventh week. With the formation of the membranous part of the interventricular septum by the end of the seventh week, the interventricular foramen is obliterated. The membranous part of the interventricular septum, derived from the fused endocardial cushions, merges with the bulbar ridges of the aorticopulmonary septum and the muscular part of the interventricular septum.

28. **C** The distal part of the arch of the aorta is derived from the left dorsal aorta; its proximal part is formed from the fourth aortic arch and the aortic sac. In this case of transposition of the great arteries, the aorta is shown arising from the right ventricle. Coarctation of the aorta almost invariably is located where the ductus arteriosus connects with the aortic arch and the descending aorta.

29. **A** The formation and subsequent fusion of the septum primum and septum secundum divide the primordial atrium into a right atrium and a left atrium. Initially, the sinus venosus opens into the dorsal wall of the primordial right atrium. By the end of the fourth week, the right horn of the sinus venosus is larger than the left. The right horn of the sinus venosus becomes incorporated into the wall of the right atrium, and the left horn forms the coronary sinus. The smooth part of the wall of the right atrium is known as the sinus venarum because it is derived from the sinus venosus.

# Skeletal and Muscular Systems

**15**

## Objectives

**Be able to:**

- Construct and label diagrams showing the early differentiation of somites.
- Describe endochondral and intramembranous bone formation.
- Construct and label diagrams showing the development of the different types of joint.
- Describe the development of a typical vertebra.
- Make simple sketches of the fetal cranium showing the bones, fontanelles, and sutures.
- Discuss briefly: achondroplasia, spina bifida occulta, cervical and lumbar ribs, acrania, and craniosynostosis.

## Five-Choice Completion Questions

**Directions:** Each of the following statements or questions is followed by five suggested responses or completions. **Select the one best answer** in each case.

1. Which of the following bones is formed by intramembranous ossification?
   A. humerus
   B. mandible
   C. hyoid
   D. occipital
   E. tibia

2. Which of the following bones is completely formed by intramembranous ossification?
   A. stapes
   B. parietal
   C. clavicle
   D. radius
   E. sphenoid

3. The most common type of accessory rib is a _____ rib.
   A. lumbar
   B. forked
   C. cervical
   D. thoracic
   E. fused

4. Myoblasts from the occipital myotomes give rise to the muscles of the
   A. eye
   B. ear
   C. neck
   D. tongue
   E. pharynx

5. The pharyngeal and laryngeal muscles develop from mesenchyme derived from the
    A. preotic myotomes
    B. occipital myotomes
    C. splanchnic mesoderm
    D. somatic mesoderm
    E. pharyngeal arches

6. Which of the following bones is *not* derived mainly from the cartilaginous viscerocranium?
    A. malleus
    B. incus
    C. stapes
    D. occipital
    E. hyoid

7. Increase in the size of the calvaria is greatest during the first _____ years.
    A. 2
    B. 3
    C. 5
    D. 7
    E. 9

8. The neonate's face is relatively small compared with the calvaria. Enlargement of the facial region during childhood mainly results from an increase in the size of the
    A. paranasal sinuses
    B. deciduous teeth
    C. nose and jaws
    D. permanent teeth
    E. brain and calvaria

9. The skeleton shows clearly on radiographs by the beginning of the _____ week.
    A. seventh
    B. ninth
    C. eleventh
    D. thirteenth
    E. fifteenth

10. Achondroplasia was diagnosed in a child. This anomaly
    A. results from a disturbance of intramembranous ossification
    B. is an autosomal recessive condition
    C. is an autosomal dominant condition
    D. is an uncommon cause of dwarfism
    E. increases with maternal age

11. Congenital torticollis was diagnosed in an infant whose head was tilted to the right with the chin turned to the left. Which of the following is involved?
    A. right sternocleidomastoid muscle
    B. left trapezius muscle
    C. fusion of the cervical vertebrae
    D. vertebral anomalies
    E. absence of right pectoralis major muscle

12. A 26-year-old female patient complained of weakness and loss of sensation on the medial side of her arm. X ray examination of the neck and thorax revealed the presence of a cervical rib. Cervical rib
    A. occurs only on one side of the neck
    B. may compress the brachial plexus
    C. is found in 5 to 10% of the population
    D. is attached to an upper cervical vertebra
    E. is the most common type of accessory rib

# Answers and Explanations

1. **B**   The mandible forms almost entirely by intramembranous ossification. Some endochondral ossification occurs in a small portion of the anterior part of the mandible and at its condyle. The mesenchyme in the mandibular process of the first pharyngeal arch condenses around the first arch cartilage to form a dense fibromembranous tissue; this undergoes intramembranous ossification as the cartilage degenerates. Hence, endochondral ossification does not occur in the cartilage, as one might expect.

2. **B**   The parietal and other flat bones of the neurocranium develop by intramembranous ossification. The clavicle begins to develop by intramembranous ossification, but later it develops growth cartilages at each end that give rise to most of the bone.

3. **A**   Rudimentary lumbar ribs are the most common type of accessory rib, but they usually are of no clinical significance. Cervical ribs are attached to the seventh cervical vertebra. They may be unilateral or bilateral, complete or incomplete. A cervical rib usually causes no symptoms; however, the subclavian artery and the inferior part of the brachial plexus may cross over the cervical rib. In these cases, the rib may exert pressure on these structures and give rise to pain and/or muscular atrophy in the upper limb.

4. **D**   There initially are four occipital somites and, hence, four occipital myotomes. The first pair of somites disappears, and the myotomes of the others give rise to mesenchyme that forms the tongue muscles. When the myoblasts that give rise to these muscles migrate to the tongue, they carry their nerve supply with them.

5. **E**   The mesenchyme that gives rise to the myoblasts that form the pharyngeal and laryngeal muscles is derived from the fourth and sixth pharyngeal arches. These muscles are innervated by the vagus nerve (CN X), the nerve that supplies these arches.

6. **D**   The occipital bone is derived mainly by ossification of the dorsal part of the cartilaginous neurocranium. The part of this bone superior to the highest nuchal line develops by intramembranous ossification. The cartilaginous viscerocranium consists of the cartilaginous skeleton of the first two pairs of pharyngeal arches. Parts of the cartilages in these arches undergo endochondral ossification to form bone (e.g., the styloid process of the temporal bone).

7. **A**   Growth of the calvaria is rapid during infancy, especially during the first 2 years. This growth is related primarily to the extensive development of the brain during this period. The calvaria normally increases slightly in capacity until 15 or 16 years of age.

8. **A**   Enlargement of the frontal and facial regions of the postnatal cranium results mainly from the increase in size of the paranasal sinuses. These air sinuses develop during the late fetal period and infancy as small diverticula of the lateral walls of the nasal cavities. During childhood, the sinuses also extend into the maxilla, ethmoid, frontal, and sphenoid bones. This causes enlargement of the face. There is concurrent development of the jaws as the teeth develop and erupt.

9. **E**   Although the fetal skeleton may be visualized earlier than 15 weeks on radiographs, it usually is not clearly displayed until after the fourteenth week. X-ray investigations often raise concerns about the hazards of ionizing radiation. Embryos are particularly radiosensitive during the period of organogenesis. The fetal gonads and the brain are radiosensitive throughout the fetal period. Because of this, ultrasound scans of the uterus often are used to diagnose twins, locate the placenta, and study the fetal cranium. There is no increased incidence of congenital abnormalities or evidence of tissue damage caused by sound energy in infants of mothers who have undergone sonography.

10. **C**   Achondroplasia is an autosomal dominant disorder. It is the most common cause of dwarfism and occurs with a frequency of about 1:10,000 births. The limbs are short, the head is

relatively large, and there is thoracic kyphosis with protrusion of the abdomen. Disturbance of endochondral ossification at the epiphysial cartilage plates results in the short limbs. The rate of achondroplasia increases with paternal age. This anomaly results from a mutation in the FGFR3 gene on chromosome 4p.

11. **A**  The right sternocleidomastoid muscle is shortened, resulting in the ear being closer to the shoulder on the affected side and the chin rotated toward the opposite side. The cause is not known. Because torticollis has been observed in infants delivered by cesarean section, it has been

suggested that factors other than birth trauma may be involved. Absence of the sternal part of the pectoralis major muscle is not uncommon, but it is unrelated to congenital torticollis.

12. **B**  Cervical rib occurs in 0.5 to 1% of the population. It is attached to the seventh cervical vertebra and may be unilateral or bilateral. The most common type of accessory rib is a lumbar rib. Pressure of the cervical rib on the inferior trunk of the brachial plexus and the subclavian artery often produces clinical symptoms, such as numbness and ischemic pain in the upper limb.

# *Five-Choice Association Questions*

**Directions:** Each group of questions below consists of a numbered list of descriptive words or phrases accompanied by a diagram with certain parts indicated by letters or by a list of lettered headings. For each numbered word or phrase, **select the lettered part or heading** that matches it correctly and then insert the letter in the space to the right of the appropriate number. Sometimes more than one numbered word or phrase may be correctly matched to the same lettered part or heading.

A. Centrum
B. Epiphysial plate
C. Frontal bone
D. Anterior fontanelle
E. Cartilaginous viscerocranium

1. _____ Closes during the second year
2. _____ Forms by intramembranous ossification
3. _____ Partly within the pharyngeal arches
4. _____ Growth of long bones
5. _____ Primary ossification center
6. _____ Styloid process

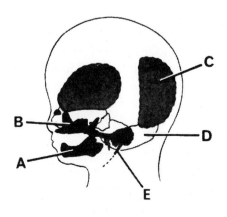

7. _____ Associated with the first pharyngeal arch cartilage
8. _____ Part of the cartilaginous viscerocranium
9. _____ Forms in the maxillary prominence of the first pharyngeal arch
10. _____ Part of the cartilaginous neurocranium
11. _____ Forms in the mandibular prominence of the first pharyngeal arch
12. _____ Part of the membranous neurocranium

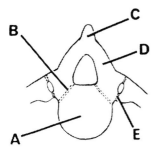

13. _____ Articulates with centrum
14. _____ Neurocentral joint
15. _____ Replaced by a synovial joint
16. _____ Centrum
17. _____ Its cartilage is ossified during infancy
18. _____ Disappears during childhood

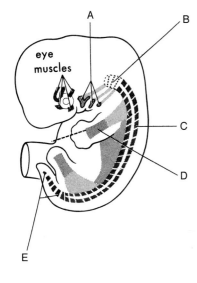

19. _____ Form the tongue muscles
20. _____ Normally regress during the eighth week
21. _____ Form the scalene muscles
22. _____ Give rise to the muscles of mastication
23. _____ Muscles originate from somites

## Answers and Explanations

1. **D**  The anterior fontanelle, located where the two parietal bones and the halves of the frontal bone meet, usually closes about the middle of the second year. Palpation of this fontanelle during infancy gives information about ossification of the cranium and intracranial pressure.

2. **C**  The frontal bone, part of the membranous neurocranium, develops by intramembranous ossification from two primary centers. The halves of the frontal bone begin to fuse during the second year, and the frontal (metopic) suture usually is obliterated by the eighth year.

3. **E**  The ends of the cartilaginous rods in the first and second pairs of pharyngeal arches reach the ventral surface of the neurocranium in the region of the developing ears. Later, they undergo endochondral ossification to form the lesser horns and the superior part of the body of the hyoid bone.

4. **B**  During the later stages of postnatal bone growth, the mass of cartilage between the diaphysis and epiphysis decreases in thickness to form a comparatively thin cartilage, the epiphysial cartilage plate. This plate is of importance for growth of long bones. At the termination of growth in the bone, the epiphysial plate disappears and the epiphysis unites with the diaphysis.

5. **A**  Most of the body of a typical vertebra (thoracic and lumbar) is ossified from a primary center, the centrum, which appears during the eighth week. At birth, the bone of the centrum is separated from the separate halves of the vertebral arch of cartilage by the neurocentral joints.

6. **E**  The styloid process of the temporal bone develops by endochondral ossification of part of the dorsal end of the cartilage of the second

pharyngeal arch. The cartilages of the first two pairs of pharyngeal arches constitute the cartilaginous viscerocranium.

7. **A** Development of the mandible is associated with the cartilage of the first pharyngeal arch. As this cartilage degenerates, the condensed mesenchyme near it undergoes intramembranous ossification to form the mandible.

8. **E** The styloid process of the temporal bone and the malleus, incus, and stapes are derived from the cartilaginous viscerocranium.

9. **B** The maxilla forms in the maxillary prominence of the first pharyngeal arch by intramembranous ossification. It is part of the membranous viscerocranium, as are the mandible, zygomatic, and squamous temporal bones.

10. **D** The occipital bone ossifies partly by endochondral ossification of the posterior part of the cartilaginous neurocranium. This plate of cartilage forms in the base of the developing cranium (skull) by the fusion of several paired cartilages.

11. **A** The mandible is the part of the membranous viscerocranium that develops mainly by intramembranous ossification around the degenerating cartilage of the first pharyngeal arch.

12. **C** The parietal and other flat bones of the cranium are parts of the membranous neurocranium that develop by intramembranous ossification. At birth, they are separated by connective tissue sutures.

13. **D** Each half of the vertebral arch (a lamina), is ossified from a primary ossification center. At birth, the laminae are separated from each other dorsally by cartilage and from the centrum by the cartilaginous neurocentral joints. These joints disappear when the vertebral arch fuses with the centrum (usually about the fifth year). The laminae of the vertebral arch fuse during the first year; failure of this fusion to occur results in spina bifida occulta.

14. **B** As stated above, the neurocentral joints are located between the centrum and the vertebral

arch. In the superior cervical vertebrae, the centra unite with the vertebral arches about the third year, but in the inferior lumbar vertebrae, union is not completed until the sixth year.

15. **E** The ribs are connected to the costal processes of thoracic vertebrae at costovertebral joints; these are the plain type of synovial joint. As the ribs and vertebrae ossify, joints develop between the tubercles of the ribs and the transverse processes of the vertebrae.

16. **A** The major part of the body of a typical vertebra is formed by the centrum. It is ossified from a primary center that appears dorsal to the notochord. The centrum occasionally is ossified from bilateral primary centers.

17. **C** The vertebrae form by the ossification of cartilaginous bone models. Primary centers appear during the early fetal period — one in each half of the vertebral arch and one in the centrum. At birth, the ossified halves of the vertebral arch are still separated from each other by cartilage. This cartilage is ossified during the first year.

18. **B** The vertebral arch during infancy and early childhood is separated from the bone of the centrum by persistent bilateral zones of cartilage (neurocentral joints). These two lateral zones are ossified during the fifth and sixth years.

19. **B** The first pair of four occipital myotomes degenerate. Myoblasts from the remaining three myotomes migrate from the occipital region to the floor of the pharynx and form the striated muscles of the tongue, with the exception of the palatoglossus muscle. The hypoglossal nerve (CN XII) supplies all the muscles of the tongue except for the palatoglossus muscle, which is supplied by the pharyngeal branch of the vagus nerve (CN X).

20. **E** The paired somites begin to differentiate from the paraxial mesoderm in a craniocaudal sequence during the third week. By the end of the fifth week, 42 to 44 pairs of somites are present. The coccygeal somites regress with the tail-like caudal eminence during the eighth week.

21. **C**  Myoblasts from the cervical myotomes form the scalene muscles, as well as the prevertebral, geniohyoid, and infrahyoid muscles.

22. **A**  Myoblasts from the pharyngeal arches migrate to form the muscles of mastication (temporal, masseter, and medial and lateral pterygoids). The muscles of facial expression, as well as those of the pharynx and larynx, are also formed from the myoblasts of the pharyngeal arches. Muscles derived from any one of the pharyngeal arches retain the nerve supply of that particular arch; that is, the trigeminal nerve (CN V) innervates the muscles of mastication, as well as other muscles (mylohyoid, anterior belly of digastric, tensor tympani, tensor veli palatini) that are derived from the first pharyngeal arch. The facial nerve (CN VII), which is the second pharyngeal arch nerve, innervates the muscles of facial expression.

23. **D**  The limb muscles are derived from the somites. Grafting and gene targeting studies in mammals indicate that the precursor myogenic cells in limb buds originate from the somites. These cells are first located in the ventral part of the dermomyotome and are epithelial in nature. Following mesenchymal-epithelial transformation, the cells then migrate into the primordium of the limb.

# Limbs

**16**

## Objectives

Be able to:

- Define and illustrate the apical ectodermal ridge.
- Discuss the molecular mechanisms underlying normal and abnormal development of the limbs.
- Describe the development of the bones and muscles of the limbs.
- Describe the effects of teratogens on limb development.
- Construct and label diagrams showing rotation of the limbs.
- Discuss and illustrate the development of the dermatomal patterns of the limbs.

## Five-Choice Completion Questions

**Directions:** Each of the following statements or questions is followed by five suggested responses or completions. **Select the one best answer** in each case.

1. Teratogens acting after the _____ week do not cause severe limb defects.
   - A. fourth
   - B. fifth
   - C. sixth
   - D. seventh
   - E. eighth

2. The apical ectodermal ridge (AER)
   - A. first appears in the lower limb bud
   - B. is responsible for the formation of dermatomes
   - C. expresses fibroblast growth factors (FGFs)
   - D. initiates limb rotation
   - E. is induced by the ZPA

3. Which of the following bones develop by endochondral ossification?
   - A. clavicle
   - B. occipital
   - C. sphenoid
   - D. frontal
   - E. mandible

4. Which of the following bones develops by intramembranous ossification?
   - A. humerus
   - B. ulna
   - C. radius
   - D. phalanges
   - E. clavicle

5. Congenital clubfoot was diagnosed in a child. In this condition, which of the following statements is correct?
   - A. The bones have fused.
   - B. The talus is involved.
   - C. The foot is everted.
   - D. It is more common in females.
   - E. The calcaneus is absent.

6. With respect to congenital dislocation of the hip, all of the following are correct *except*:
   A. It is more common in females than in males.  D. It occurs in about 1:1500 births.
   B. Dislocation of the hip occurs in utero.  E. Hereditary factors are involved.
   C. The acetabulum is underdeveloped.

7. For a teratogen to cause absence of the hand, it would have to act before the end of the _____ week.
   A. fifth  D. eighth
   B. sixth  E. ninth
   C. seventh

8. With respect to polydactyly, all of the following are correct *except*:
   A. Supernumerary digits are common.
   B. It is inherited as a dominant trait.
   C. In the hand, the extra digit is most commonly central.
   D. In the foot, the extra digit is usually located on the lateral side.
   E. The extra digit usually lacks proper muscular development.

9. Ossification of the long bones of the limbs begins in the _____ week.
   A. sixth  D. ninth
   B. seventh  E. tenth
   C. eighth

10. A full-term infant was born with varying degrees of "webbing" between the fingers. It was diagnosed as a cutaneous syndactyly which
    A. is an uncommon anomaly
    B. occurs more frequently in the hand than in the foot
    C. is inherited as a dominant or recessive trait
    D. results from failure of the digital rays to degenerate
    E. is caused by the breakdown of mesenchymal tissue between digital rays

## Answers and Explanations

1. **C**  By the end of the sixth week, the digital rays of the fingers and toes are differentiated; hence, after this period, teratogenic substances (e.g., drugs) are unable to produce major congenital anomalies (e.g., meromelia — partial absence of a limb).

2. **C**  The AER first appears at the distal end of the upper limb bud. It expresses various fibroblast growth factors which regulate limb outgrowth (progress zone) and distal patterning. The AER is induced by mesoderm. The ZPA is located on the posterior margin of the limb bud. It controls anteroposterior patterning of the limb. The AER is not responsible for dermatome formation and rotation of the limb. Injury to the AER results in severe limb defects.

3. **C**  In general, the bones of the base of the cranium (chondrocranium), like the long bones of the skeleton, ossify in cartilage (endochondral ossification). Mesenchymal condensation occurs and is replaced by a hyaline cartilage model. Most bones are formed by this process. The clavicle, mandible, and the flat bones of the calvaria (neurocranium) develop by intramembranous ossification.

4. **E**  All of the limb bones form by endochondral ossification. Mesenchymal models of the bones form, and chondrification results in cartilage models. Later, bone forms. Between the sixth and seventh week, the clavicle begins its formation by intramembranous ossification. It is the first bone to ossify in the body.

5. **B** Any deformity of the foot that involves the talus (ankle bone) is known as a clubfoot. In talipes equinovarus, which is the most common type of clubfoot and far more common in males than in females, the sole is turned medially and the foot is inverted. It is believed that both hereditary factors and in utero compression of the fetal lower limbs are responsible for this deformity.

6. **B** Dislocation of the hip almost always occurs after birth. Acetabular insufficiency, laxity of the joint, and hereditary factors usually are involved in the development of this deformity. A higher risk of occurrence exists among siblings because joint laxity often is dominantly inherited.

7. **A** The potent teratogen (thalidomide) known to cause limb defects did not induce absence of the hand when it was ingested later than thirty-three days after the last normal menstrual period. During the sixth to eighth week, only minor limb defects (e.g., hypoplasia of the thumb) can be produced by a teratogenic agent.

8. **C** In polydactyly, one or more extra digits may be present. The condition is a dominant trait and usually runs in families. If the hand is affected, the extra digit is most commonly lateral or medial rather than central. In the foot,

the extra digit is usually located on the lateral side. The extra digit is often incompletely formed and lacks proper muscular development.

9. **B** Ossification of the long bones in the limbs begins in the seventh week from primary ossification centers in the middle of the cartilaginous models of the long bones. Cartilage formation in the limbs begins during the fifth week from the mesenchymal models of the bones, and by the end of the sixth week the entire limb skeleton is cartilaginous.

10. **C** Cutaneous syndactyly (simple webbing of the digits) is the most common limb anomaly. This defect is found in about 1:3000 newborns. In more serious cases, there is fusion of the digits. It occurs more frequently in the foot than in the hand. Syndactyly is inherited as a simple dominant or simple recessive trait. Cutaneous syndactyly results when the web between two or more digital rays fails to degenerate. Breakdown of the interdigital tissue normally occurs by the end of the eighth week. Fusion of the bones (osseous syndactyly) occurs when the notches between the digital rays fail to develop during the seventh week. The digital rays are formed by mesenchymal condensations and represent the primordia of the future digits.

# Five-Choice Association Questions

**Directions:** Each group of questions below consists of a numbered list of descriptive words or phrases accompanied by a diagram with certain parts indicated by letters or by a list of lettered headings. For each numbered word or phrase, **select the lettered part or heading** that matches it correctly, and then insert the letter in the space to the right of the appropriate number. Sometimes more than one numbered word or phrase may be correctly matched to the same lettered part or heading.

A. Upper limb
B. Apical ectodermal ridge
C. Somites
D. Meromelia
E. Lower limb

1. _____ Partial absence of a limb
2. _____ Limb muscles
3. _____ Rotates medially
4. _____ Rotates laterally
5. _____ Exerts an inductive influence
6. _____ Thalidomide ingestion

A. Dermatome
B. Phocomelia
C. Digital rays
D. End of fourth week
E. Amelia

7. _____ Condensations of mesenchyme
8. _____ Lower limb bud
9. _____ Area of skin supplied by a spinal nerve
10. _____ Absence of the limbs
11. _____ Type of meromelia

---

## Answers and Explanations

1. **D** Meromelia (from Greek *meros,* part, and *melos,* extremity) is the term now used to classify all limb defects that involve partial absence of a limb or limbs — including *hemimelia* (absence of all or part of the distal half of a limb) and *phocomelia* (absence of the proximal part of a limb or limbs).

2. **C** The limb muscles develop from mesenchyme that is derived from mesenchyme in the myotome regions of the somites. Following mesenchymal-epithelial transformation, the muscle forming cells — *myoblasts* — migrate into the primordia of the limbs.

3. **E** The developing lower limbs rotate medially through almost 90 degrees. As a result, the knees face anterolaterally.

4. **A** The developing upper limbs rotate laterally through 90 degrees on their longitudinal axes; as a result, the elbows face dorsally or posteriorly in an embryo at the end of the eighth week.

5. **B** The apical ectodermal ridge (AER) is a thickened, epithelial plaque at the distal end of each limb bud. The AER exerts an inductive influence on the limb mesenchyme that initiates growth and development of the limbs. There is no further elaboration of distal structures (hands and fingers) if the ridge is removed experimentally.

6. **D** Meromelia (partial absence of the limbs) commonly was observed in the infants of mothers who ingested thalidomide during the most critical period of limb development (fourth and fifth weeks).

7. **C** The digital rays are condensations of mesenchyme in the hand and foot plates that indicate where the digits are developing.

8. **D** The lower limb buds appear at the end of the fourth week as ventrolateral outgrowths of the body wall.

9. **A** A dermatome is the area of skin supplied by a single spinal nerve and its spinal ganglion (dorsal root ganglion).

10. **E** Amelia refers to absence of a limb(s). This condition resulted when thalidomide was ingested by pregnant women early in the fourth week after fertilization.

11. **B** Phocomelia is a type of meromelia (partial absence of the limbs). In this type of meromelia, the limbs have a flipper-like appearance. The term "phocomelia" is not commonly used; meromelia is the preferred term for all defects involving partial absence of a limb(s).

# Nervous System

## Objectives

Be able to:

- Construct and label diagrams showing early development of the nervous system (CNS).
- Define neural plate, neural groove, neural folds, neural crest, neuropores, and primary and secondary brain vesicles.
- Make a simple diagram showing the development of neurons and neuroglial cells.
- Construct and label diagrams showing the brain flexures and indicating the adult derivatives of the walls and cavities of the forebrain, midbrain, and hindbrain.
- Prepare sketches showing the development of the pituitary gland.
- Discuss the following congenital anomalies of the CNS: meroanencephaly, microcephaly, encephalocele, cranial meningocele, Arnold-Chiari anomaly, spina bifida with meningocele, and spina bifida with meningomyelocele.

## Five-Choice Completion Questions

**Directions:** Each of the following statements or questions is followed by five suggested responses or completions. **Select the one best answer** in each case.

1. The rostral and caudal neuropores usually close during the _____ week.
   - A. third
   - B. fourth
   - C. fifth
   - D. sixth
   - E. seventh

2. The pons and cerebellum are derived from the walls of the
   - A. hindbrain
   - B. mesencephalon
   - C. myelencephalon
   - D. midbrain
   - E. metencephalon

3. A 26-year-old man with blurred vision and loss of motor skill was diagnosed with a neurological disorder relating to myelination of nerve fibers. The myelin sheaths surrounding axons in the CNS are formed by
   - A. neuroglial cells
   - B. astrocytes
   - C. oligodendrocytes
   - D. microglial cells
   - E. Schwann cells

4. Mesoderm gives rise to
   - A. ependymal cells
   - B. microglial cells
   - C. astroglia
   - D. suprarenal medulla
   - E. choroid epithelial cells

5. The neuroepithelium of the neural tube gives rise to
   A. melanocytes
   B. Schwann cells
   C. ependymal cells
   D. chromaffin cells
   E. spinal ganglion cells

6. The brain flexure that develops between the metencephalon and the myelencephalon is the _____ flexure.
   A. pontine
   B. cervical
   C. hindbrain
   D. midbrain
   E. cerebellar

7. The neurolemma and myelin sheath of a peripheral nerve fiber are formed by
   A. mesenchymal cells
   B. microglia
   C. neural cells
   D. Schwann cells
   E. neuroepithelial cells

8. The longitudinal groove in the internal surface of the developing spinal cord is called the
   A. neural groove
   B. cuneate groove
   C. sulcus limitans
   D. sulcus longitudinalis
   E. longitudinal groove

9. A patient was diagnosed with a neuromuscular disease involving neurons in the basal plate. Which of the following is derived from the basal plate?
   A. gracile nucleus
   B. pontine nucleus
   C. dorsal gray horn
   D. cuneate nucleus
   E. ventral gray horn

10. Which of the following structures is *not* a derivative of the diencephalon?
    A. thalamus
    B. adenohypophysis
    C. hypothalamus
    D. neurohypophysis
    E. epithalamus

11. The formation of myelin sheaths is largely completed by the end of the _____ period.
    A. embryonic
    B. fetal
    C. perinatal
    D. neonatal
    E. infantile

12. The pineal gland (body) develops as a diverticulum of the caudal part of the roof of the
    A. telencephalon
    B. diencephalon
    C. forebrain
    D. mesencephalon
    E. midbrain

13. The caudal end of the spinal cord at birth lies at the level of the _____ vertebra.
    A. third sacral
    B. first sacral
    C. third lumbar
    D. first lumbar
    E. twelfth thoracic

14. Which of the following may follow fetal infection with cytomegalovirus or *Toxoplasma gondii*?
    A. mental retardation
    B. hydrocephaly
    C. microcephaly
    D. microphthalmia
    E. all of the above

15. Which of the following congenital anomalies of the CNS is shown?

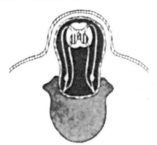

    A. spina bifida with meningocele
    B. spina bifida cystica
    C. spina bifida occulta
    D. spina bifida with myeloschisis
    E. spina bifida with meningomyelocele

16. At autopsy, a female infant was described as having a major congenital anomaly resulting from failure of the rostral neuropore to close. This condition is known as
    A. spina bifida
    B. meningocele
    C. myeloschisis
    D. meroanencephaly
    E. hydrocephalus

17. A neonate was diagnosed as having noncommunicating hydrocephalus. Which of the following might have caused this condition?
    A. Excess production of cerebrospinal fluid (CSF)
    B. Obstruction in the circulation of CSF
    C. Increased size of the head
    D. Disturbances in the resorption of CSF
    E. Failure of the neural tube to close

18. Agenesis of the corpus callosum was diagnosed in an infant. Which of the following statements about this condition is (are) correct?
    A. The cause of agenesis of the corpus callosum is not known.
    B. The corpus callosum may be partially absent.
    C. The condition may be asymptomatic.
    D. The corpus callosum may be completely absent.
    E. All of the above.

19. Most likely, induction of the neural plate is initiated by inhibition of
    A. nerve growth factor (NGF)
    B. retinoic acid
    C. bone morphogenetic proteins (BMPs)
    D. Hox genes
    E. fibroblast growth factors (FGFs)

20. The rostro-caudal axis and segmental levels of the neural tube are determined by expression of
    A. engrailed
    B. Pax
    C. TGF-$\beta$
    D. nerve growth factor
    E. Hox genes

## Answers and Explanations

1. **B** The cranial opening in the neural tube — the rostral neuropore closes at about 26 days, and the caudal neuropore closes about 2 days later. Failure of the neural folds to fuse and form the forebrain vesicle, or failure of the rostral neuropore to close, results in meroanencephaly (anencephaly). The brain is represented by a mass of largely degenerated nervous tissue. Failure of the neural folds to fuse into the neural tube in the region that gives rise to the spinal cord, or failure of the caudal neuropore to close, results in spina bifida cystica (e.g., spina bifida with meningocele).

2. **E** The walls of the metencephalon give rise to the pons and cerebellum; its cavity forms the superior part of the fourth ventricle. If you chose answer **A**, you were partly correct because the metencephalon is the rostral part of the hindbrain. Answer **E** is more specific; thus, it is the better of the two answers.

3. **C** Oligodendrocytes form the myelin sheaths in the CNS in the same way that Schwann cells form the myelin sheaths of peripheral nerve fibers. The plasma membrane of an oligodendrocyte wraps around a nerve fiber. The number of layers that are wrapped around the fiber determines the thickness of the myelin sheath. If you selected choice **A**, you were partly right because oligodendrocytes are a type of neuroglial cell. Choice **C** is more specific; thus, it is the better of the two answers.

4. **B** The microglial cells (microglia), scattered through the gray and white substance (matter) of the CNS, are derived from mesoderm. They invade the central nervous system late in fetal development. Ependymal cells, astroglia, motor neurons, and choroid epithelial cells are derived from the neuroectoderm.

5. **C** Ependymal cells, often classified as a type of neuroglial cell, are derived from the neuroepithelium of the neural tube. After the production of neuroblasts (developing neurons) has ceased, the neuroepithelial cells lining the ven-

tricles and the central canal of the spinal cord form the ependymal epithelium or ependyma. Throughout most of the ventricular surface, the ependymal cells have cilia that project into the ventricles.

6. **A** The pontine flexure causes the lateral walls of the medulla to fall outward or laterally like the pages of an opening book. This causes the roof plate to be stretched and the cavity of the hindbrain (future fourth ventricle) to become somewhat rhomboidal or diamond-shaped.

7. **D** The neurolemma (sheath of Schwann) and myelin sheath are both formed by Schwann cells, which are derived from the neural crest. These cells migrate peripherally and wrap themselves around the fibers of peripheral nerves. One Schwann cell may envelop up to 15 fibers that remain as unmyelinated fibers. Schwann cells ensheathing a single axon develop myelin between the axon and the neurolemma (neurilemma) by rotation of the Schwann cell around the axon.

8. **C** The sulcus limitans results from differential thickening of the lateral walls of the developing spinal cord. This sulcus or groove demarcates the dorsal or alar plate (lamina) from the ventral or basal plate (lamina). This regional separation is of fundamental importance because the alar and basal plates are later associated with afferent and efferent functions, respectively.

9. **E** The neurons that form the gray substance (matter) in the ventral or anterior horns of the spinal cord are derived from neuroblasts in the basal plates. The lateral gray columns of the spinal cord are also derived from the basal plates. The alar laminae form the gray columns in the dorsal horns. Axons from motor neurons of the ventral horns of the spinal cord innervate skeletal muscles.

10. **B** The adenohypophysis or glandular part of the pituitary gland is not derived from the diencephalon. It originates from the hypophysial

pouch (Rathke pouch), a diverticulum from the roof of the primordial mouth or stomodeum. The neurohypophysis is derived from the infundibulum, a downgrowth from the floor of the diencephalon.

11. **E** Myelination begins during midfetal life (16 to 20 weeks) and is largely completed by the end of the infantile period (12 to 14 months). There are exceptions to these general statements; for example, the descending motor tracts (pyramidal and rubrospinal) do not begin to acquire their myelin sheaths until full term, and the process is not complete until the end of the second year of postnatal life. There is good evidence to indicate that tracts become completely myelinated at about the time they become fully functional.

12. **B** The pineal gland develops as a midline diverticulum of the caudal part of the roof of the diencephalon. It eventually becomes a solid organ located on the roof of the mesencephalon (midbrain). When stimulated, sympathetic fibers in the pineal gland release norepinephrine.

13. **C** The caudal end of the spinal cord usually lies at the level of the third lumbar vertebra in the neonate. This is an average level; it could end as high as the second lumbar vertebra or as low as the fourth lumbar vertebra. In the embryo, the spinal cord extends the entire length of the vertebral canal. Because the vertebral column grows more rapidly than the spinal cord, the cord gradually comes to lie at relatively higher levels. Because part of the subarachnoid space extends below the spinal cord (i.e., below L3 in the neonate), CSF may be removed without damaging the cord. In the adult, the spinal cord usually ends at the inferior border of the first lumbar vertebra.

14. **E** Maternal infections (cytomegalovirus and *Toxoplasma gondii*) during the fetal period may cause all the congenital abnormalities listed. Rubella infections during the second trimester often produce effects similar to those caused by cytomegalovirus and the parasite *T. gondii,* except that the rubella virus usually causes more severe abnormalities, especially of the eyes and ears.

15. **E** If you chose **B**, you selected the second best answer; it is not as specific as choice **E** because **A** and **D** are also types of spina bifida cystica; that is, they exhibit a saccular protrusion of the spinal cord and/or the meninges.

16. **D** Failure of the rostral neuropore to close results in meroanencephaly (anencephaly), a clinical condition that is incompatible with postnatal life because only a small part of the hindbrain is present. It occurs more frequently in female infants.

17. **B** Hydrocephalus is an accumulation of CSF in the ventricular system. There are two types: communicating and noncommunicating. Obstruction in the circulation of CSF results in a noncommunicating hydrocephalus, and a communicating hydrocephalus results from either an excess production or poor resorption of CSF. Increase in the size of the ventricles causes compression and atrophy of the brain, with the head becoming progressively larger.

18. **E** The corpus callosum is the largest cerebral commissure connecting the cerebral hemispheres. It may be partially or completely absent. The cause of this condition is not known, and there is no evidence that it is inherited. Patients with agenesis of the corpus callosum often present without any symptoms and usually have average IQs. Seizures and mental deficiency are not uncommon in some people with agenesis of the corpus callosum.

19. **C** Molecular studies suggest that induction of the neural plate begins with the inhibition of BMPs in the epiblast. The inhibitory signals originate from the notochord and surrounding tissues. The other items listed are not involved in neural induction.

20. **E** Differential expression of Hox genes during neuralation specify the rostro-caudal axis and regionalization levels of the neural tube.

# *Five-Choice Association Questions*

**Directions:** Each group of questions below consists of a numbered list of descriptive words or phrases accompanied by a diagram with certain parts indicated by letters or by a list of lettered headings. For each numbered word or phrase, **select the lettered part or heading** that matches it correctly and then insert the letter in the space to the right of the appropriate number. Sometimes more than one numbered word or phrase may be correctly matched to the same lettered part or heading.

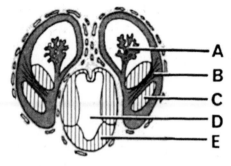

A. Neural crest cells
B. Alar plates
C. Basal plates
D. Neuroepithelium
E. Spinal ganglion cells

1. _____ Lentiform nucleus
2. _____ Invagination of pia mater
3. _____ Third ventricle
4. _____ Produces CSF
5. _____ Hypothalamus
6. _____ Internal capsule

7. _____ Gracile nuclei
8. _____ Form ventral gray columns
9. _____ Sympathetic ganglion cells
10. _____ Neuroglia
11. _____ Efferent function
12. _____ Unipolar afferent neurons

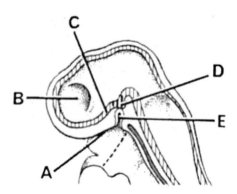

A. Telencephalon
B. Diencephalon
C. Mesencephalon
D. Metencephalon
E. Myelencephalon

13. _____ Primordium of adenohypophysis
14. _____ Gives rise to the pars nervosa
15. _____ Roof of primordial mouth cavity
16. _____ Infundibulum
17. _____ Primordium of the cerebral hemisphere
18. _____ Floor of the diencephalon

19. _____ Pons
20. _____ Olivary nuclei
21. _____ Corpus striatum
22. _____ Thalamus
23. _____ Red nuclei
24. _____ Cerebellum

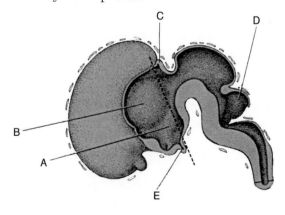

25. _____ Neurohypophysial bud
26. _____ Gives rise to the neurohypophysis
27. _____ Forms the thalamus
28. _____ Includes the mammillary bodies
29. _____ Forms the pineal gland
30. _____ Develops from the metencephalon

## Answers and Explanations

1. **C**  As the cerebral cortex differentiates, nerve fibers passing to and from it pass through the swelling — corpus striatum — in the floor of each hemisphere. Soon these fibers divide the corpus striatum into two groups of nerve cells, the caudate and lentiform nuclei.

2. **A**  The choroid plexus of the lateral ventricle is formed by an invagination of vascular pia mater — tela choroidea — on the medial side of each cerebral hemisphere. The vascular connective tissue acquires a covering layer of epithelium from the ependymal lining of the ventricle.

3. **D**  The third ventricle is formed mainly from the cavity of the diencephalon. The anterior part of the third ventricle is derived from the cavity of the telencephalon.

4. **A**  The choroid plexuses of the lateral, third, and fourth ventricles produce most of the CSF. The plexuses in the lateral ventricles are the largest and most important producers of CSF. Some CSF is formed by the pia mater on the external surface of the brain.

5. **E**  The hypothalamus arises by proliferation of neuroblasts in the ventral wall of the diencephalon. The various nuclei that develop in it are concerned with endocrine activities and homeostasis.

6. **B**  As the cerebral cortex differentiates, fibers passing to and from it pass through the corpus striatum; this fiber pathway is the internal capsule. Projection fibers concentrated in the internal capsule fan out to form the corona radiata in the medullary center. Because of its adaptation to the contours of the masses of gray substance (matter) in the brain, the internal capsule develops an anterior limb, a genu, and a posterior limb, as seen on horizontal section.

7. **B**  The gracile and cuneate nuclei develop from neuroblasts that migrate from the alar plates into the marginal zone of the myelencephalon. These nuclei are associated with correspondingly named tracts that enter the medulla from the spinal cord.

8. **C**  The basal plates of the neural tube give rise to the ventral and lateral gray columns of nerve cells in the spinal cord. Axons of the ventral horn cells grow out of the spinal cord and form the ventral roots of spinal nerves.

9. **A**  Sympathetic ganglion cells are derived from neuroblasts that differentiate from neural crest cells. Some sympathetic neuroblasts migrate to the suprarenal glands where they differentiate into chromaffin cells of the suprarenal medulla.

10. **D**  Some neuroepithelial cells of the neural tube differentiate into glioblasts (spongioblasts). These cells give rise to oligodendroblasts and astroblasts, which eventually become oligodendrocytes and astrocytes. Oligodendrocytes are concerned with the formation of myelin sheaths within the central nervous system, and astrocytes provide nutrition and general support to the developing neurons. The formation of glial cells continues into adult life.

11. **C**  Neuroepithelial cells in the basal plates of the developing neural tube give rise to neurons (e.g., the motor neurons in the ventral horns of the spinal córd) that are concerned with efferent activities.

12. **E**  The unipolar spinal (dorsal root) ganglion cells arise by differentiation of neural crest cells, but they are not unipolar neurons. First bipolar neuroblasts form and then their processes unite to form unipolar neurons. The central process of this T-shaped axon grows into the spinal cord to form part of a dorsal root; the peripheral process forms part of the dorsal root, which joins the ventral root to form a mixed spinal nerve.

13. **E**  The primordium of the adenohypophysis is the hypophysial (Rathke) pouch, a diverticulum from the ectodermal roof of the primordial mouth cavity. This diverticulum soon contacts the infundibulum, the primordium of the neurohypophysis.

14. **D**  The infundibulum gives rise to the neurohypophysis. The infundibulum appears as a diverticulum of the floor of the diencephalon.

Later, nerve fibers from the hypothalamus grow into the developing pars nervosa of the pituitary gland.

15. **A** The epithelial roof of the primordial mouth cavity (stomodeum) is derived from ectoderm. As the head folds and the pharyngeal arches form during the fourth week, the surface ectoderm becomes depressed to form the primordial mouth cavity in the center of the facial primordia. The hypophysial pouch develops as a dorsal diverticulum of the oral ectoderm.

16. **D** The infundibulum gives rise to the neurohypophysis or pars nervosa of the pituitary gland. As the posterior pituitary develops, the neuroepithelial cells in the wall of the infundibulum proliferate and differentiate into pituicytes.

17. **B** The lateral diverticulum of the telencephalon gives rise to the right cerebral hemisphere. As it expands, it covers the diencephalon, midbrain, and hindbrain. It eventually meets the other hemisphere in the midline, flattening their medial surfaces.

18. **C** The floor of the diencephalon gives rise to the infundibulum (the primordium of the neurohypophysis) and the mammillary bodies. The infundibulum gives rise to the median eminence, the infundibular stem, and the pars nervosa. The infundibulum initially has a thin wall, but its distal end soon becomes thickened as the neuroepithelial cells proliferate. These cells later differentiate into pituicytes.

19. **D** The pons is derived from the metencephalon. Nerve fibers that connect the cerebral and cerebellar cortices with the spinal cord pass through the marginal layer of the ventral region of the metencephalon. These fibers form a robust band of nerve fibers crossing to the other side. This accounts for the name *pons,* a Latin word meaning a bridge. The walls of the metencephalon form the pons and cerebellum, and its cavity forms the superior part of the fourth ventricle.

20. **E** The olivary nuclei in the rostral part of the myelencephalon (open part of the medulla) are derived from neuroblasts that migrate from the alar plates.

21. **A** The corpus striatum appears as a prominent swelling in the floor of each cerebral hemisphere. The hemispheres develop from lateral diverticula of the telencephalon. Because of the presence of the corpus striatum in the floor of the hemisphere, the floor expands more slowly than the thin cortical walls. Consequently, the cerebral hemispheres assume a **C** shape.

22. **B** The thalamus develops from a swelling on each side of the lateral wall of the diencephalon. As the thalamic swellings enlarge, they bulge into the cavity of the diencephalon (developing third ventricle), reducing it to a narrow cavity. The thalamic swellings often meet and fuse in the midline, forming the interthalamic adhesion (massa intermedia), which bridges the cavity of the third ventricle.

23. **C** The red nuclei of the midbrain are derived from neuroblasts that arise from the basal plates of the mesencephalon. The basal plates also give rise to the nuclei of the third and fourth cranial nerves and to neurons of the reticular nuclei.

24. **D** The cerebellum develops from symmetrical thickenings of the rostrodorsal parts of the alar plates of the metencephalon. The cerebellar swellings bulge into the cavity of the metencephalon (future fourth ventricle). These primordia eventually fuse and overgrow the rostral half of the fourth ventricle and overlap the pons and medulla.

25. **E** The neurohypophysial bud develops as a ventral diverticulum of the floor of the diencephalon. This bud enlarges to form the infundibulum, primordium of the median eminence, infundibular stem, and pars nervosa of the pituitary gland.

26. **E** The pituitary gland develops from two sources: an upgrowth of the ectodermal roof of the stomodeum and a downgrowth from the neuroectoderm of the diencephalon, known as the infundibulum or neurohypophysial bud. The neurohypophysis, which consists of the

median eminence, infundibular stem, and pars nervosa of the pituitary gland, is derived from the infundibulum.

27. **B** The thalamus develops rapidly in the lateral walls of the third ventricle, reducing it to a narrow cleft. In most brains, the thalami meet and fuse in the midline, forming a bridge of gray matter — the interthalamic adhesion — across the third ventricle.

28. **A** The mammillary bodies are located on the ventral surface of the hypothalamus. The hypothalamus arises by proliferation of neuroblasts in the lateral walls of the third ventricle. It is separated from the thalamus by a shallow groove, the hypothalamic sulcus.

29. **C** The pineal gland develops as a median diverticulum from the caudal part of the roof the diencephalon. It is converted into a solid cone-shaped gland by cellular proliferation.

30. **D** The cerebellum develops from the walls of the metencephalon. The pons also arises from the metencephalon. The cerebellum arises bilaterally from the dorsal parts of the alar plates. The cerebellar primordia enlarge, projecting into the fourth ventricle and eventually fuse in the median plane to form the vermis.

# Eye and Ear

**18**

## Objectives

Be able to:

- Construct and label diagrams showing early development of the eyes.
- Define optic sulci, optic vesicles, optic stalks, retinal fissures, optic cups, lens placodes, lens pits, and lens vesicles.
- Describe the development of the retina, ciliary body, and iris, using labeled sketches.
- Write brief notes on the formation of the lens, choroid, sclera, cornea, and optic nerve.
- Describe the development of the internal ear, middle ear, and external ear.
- Define otic placode, otic pit, otic vesicle, endolymphatic duct and sac, spiral organ, and semicircular ducts.
- Discuss the embryological basis of the following congenital anomalies: coloboma, glaucoma, cataract, and deafness.

## Five-Choice Completion Questions

**Directions:** Each of the following statements or questions is followed by five suggested responses or completions. **Select the one best answer** in each case.

1. Which of the following structures has a dual embryological origin?
   - A. iris
   - B. lens
   - C. cornea
   - D. primary vitreous humor
   - E. retina

2. Which of the following structures is derived from surface ectoderm?
   - A. choroid
   - B. bony labyrinth
   - C. extrinsic eye muscles
   - D. membranous labyrinth
   - E. sclera

3. Structures derived from the surface ectoderm include the
   - A. lens
   - B. otic vesicle
   - C. external acoustic meatus
   - D. corneal epithelium
   - E. all the above

4. The epithelium of the iris develops from the
   - A. inner layer of the rim of the optic cup
   - B. outer layer of the rim of the optic cup
   - C. both layers of the optic cup
   - D. mesenchyme near the rim of the optic cup
   - E. mesenchyme between the lens and the cornea

5. The inner, nonpigmented part of the ciliary epithelium is continuous with the
   A. neural layer of the retina
   B. sphincter of the pupil
   C. pigmented epithelium of the retina
   D. anterior surface of the iris
   E. corneal epithelium

6. The choroid is derived from the
   A. mesoderm surrounding the eye primordium
   B. loose mesenchyme near the optic cup
   C. mesenchyme from the occipital myotomes
   D. mesenchyme between the sclera and pigmented layer of the retina
   E. mesenchyme from the first pair of pharyngeal arches

7. Cellular components of the retina derived from the inner layer of the optic cup include
   A. rod cells
   B. ganglion cells
   C. neuroglial cells
   D. bipolar cells
   E. all the above

8. During examination of the eyes of a neonate, one pupil was pear-shaped owing to a defect in the iris. What is the most likely cause of this typical coloboma of the iris?
   A. genetic factors
   B. rubella virus
   C. toxoplasmosis
   D. radiation
   E. cytomegalovirus

9. You examine a neonate and diagnose congenital heart disease. You also observe bilateral cataracts. During discussions with the infant's mother, you learn that she had a fever, sore throat, and rash on her face, body, and limbs shortly after her first missed menstrual period. She also recalled taking some tranquilizers and sedatives during early pregnancy to settle her nerves and help her sleep. What do you think would be the most likely cause of the congenital anomalies you have detected in her baby?
   A. measles (rubeola)
   B. congenital galactosemia
   C. teratogenic drugs
   D. influenza
   E. none of the above

10. The otic vesicle (otocyst) gives rise to the
    A. saccule
    B. utricle
    C. cochlear duct
    D. endolymphatic sac
    E. all of the above

11. An inferior notch — coloboma of the iris — was detected in an infant. This condition probably is caused by
    A. disturbance in the development of the lower eyelid
    B. defective closure of the retinal fissure
    C. congenital glaucoma
    D. failure of the mesenchyme surrounding the optic cup to differentiate
    E. degeneration of the pupillary membrane

12. Physical examination of a neonate revealed that the external acoustic meatus is atretic. This condition is the result of which of the following?
    A. Otic pit did not form.
    B. Development of the first pharyngeal pouch is affected.
    C. Meatal plug failed to canalize.

D. Auricular hillocks did not develop.

E. Tubotympanic recess has degenerated.

13. Congenital cataract was diagnosed in an infant born to a mother who had contracted rubella infection during pregnancy. The transcription factor associated with lens formation is
   A. lens-specific maf (L-maf)
   B. zinc finger Y (ZFY)
   C. Sonic hedgehog (Shh)
   D. epidermal growth factor (EGF)
   E. notch

## *Answers and Explanations*

1. **C**  The cornea has a dual origin: the stratified squamous, nonkeratinizing epithelium is derived from the surface ectoderm; the substantia propria and other parts of the cornea are derived from mesoderm. Muscles usually are derived from mesoderm. The dilator and sphincter pupillae muscles of the iris are exceptions; they are derived from the neuroectoderm of the outer layer of the optic cup. The lens is derived from ectoderm, and the iris develops from the optic cup neural crest cells. The primary vitreous humor is derived from mesenchymal cells of neural crest origin.

2. **D**  The membranous labyrinth is derived from the otic vesicle (otocyst), which develops from an invagination of the surface ectoderm. The otic vesicle soon loses its connection with the surface (future skin).

3. **E**  All these structures are derived from the surface ectoderm. The lens develops from the lens vesicle; the otic vesicle gives rise to the membranous labyrinth; the external acoustic meatus develops from the first pharyngeal groove; and the corneal epithelium arises directly from the surface ectoderm. Other parts of the cornea are derived from mesoderm.

4. **C**  The double-layered, pigmented epithelium of the iris develops from the inner and outer layers of the rim of the optic cup. Because this epithelium is continuous with the ciliary epithelium and the retina, it often is wrongly assumed to be homologous only to the pigmented layers of these structures derived from the outer layer of the optic cup.

5. **A**  The ciliary epithelium is composed of two layers of cells derived from the continuation of the two layers of the retina. The cells of the inner, nonpigmented portion of the ciliary epithelium are continuous with the neural layer of the retina. The cells become heavily pigmented, however, in the iridial portion of the retina.

6. **D**  Three of these answers are correct (**A**, **B**, and **D**) but **D** is the best answer because it is the most specific. The mesenchyme surrounding the optic cup differentiates into an inner vascular layer, the choroid, and an outer fibrous layer, the sclera.

7. **E**  All these cells are derived from the inner layer of the optic cup. The rod photoreceptor cells are more numerous than the cone photoreceptors. The bipolar cells are true neurons interposed between the photoreceptor cells and the ganglion cells. The inner layers of the retina, in particular, contain neuroglial cells similar to those in the gray matter of the brain.

8. **A**  Most cases of coloboma of the iris are genetically determined with dominant transmission. Some colobomas are associated with maternal infections (including rubella and toxoplasmosis), and it is possible that these and other teratogenic factors may produce colobomas because their development can be induced experimentally in animals. The embryological basis of a typical coloboma of the iris is failure of the retinal fissure on the inferior surface of the optic cup to close. Closure of this fissure typically occurs during the sixth week.

9. **E** None of the factors listed probably caused the anomalies exhibited by the infant. The most likely cause of these abnormalities was a maternal rubella (German measles) infection during early pregnancy. Infection of the embryo by rubeola does not cause birth defects. Rubeola should not be confused with rubella. The infant exhibited two of the common abnormalities of the *congenital rubella syndrome* (congenital heart defects and cataracts). Congenital galactosemia could produce the cataracts, but this is an uncommon cause. Tranquilizers are not known to cause anomalies, and thalidomide is the only sedative known to be teratogenic. Influenza is not known to cause congenital anomalies.

10. **E** All these structures are derived from the otic vesicle (otocyst). The cochlear duct contains the spiral organ (of Corti), the receptor of auditory stimuli. The other parts of the membranous labyrinth, derived from the otic vesicle, contain sensory areas of the vestibular system.

11. **B** Coloboma of the iris is caused by a defect in the closure of the retinal (optic) fissure. This typically occurs during the sixth week. Coloboma of the iris often is associated with other ocular defects. Coloboma of the eyelid is probably caused by a localized disturbance during development of the eyelid.

12. **C** Atresia of the external acoustic meatus canal is a relatively common condition. It often is unilateral and associated with abnormalities of the auricle. Failure of the meatal plug of the first pharyngeal groove to canalize leads to atresia of the external acoustic meatus. This anomaly usually results from autosomal dominant inheritance.

13. **A** Lens formation involves expression of L-maf and other transcription factors in the lens placode and vesicle. The other listed signaling factors have not been implicated in lens development.

# Five-Choice Association Questions

**Directions:** Each group of questions below consists of a numbered list of descriptive words or phrases accompanied by a diagram with certain parts indicated by letters or by a list of lettered headings. For each numbered word or phrase, **select the lettered part or heading** that matches it correctly and then insert the letter in the space to the right of the appropriate number. Sometimes more than one numbered word or phrase may be correctly matched to the same lettered part or heading.

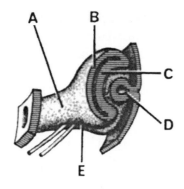

A. Scleral venous sinus
B. Optic nerve
C. Corneal epithelium
D. Central artery of retina
E. Pupillary membrane

1. _____ Becomes pigmented layer of the retina
2. _____ Retinal fissure
3. _____ Becomes specialized for sensitivity to light
4. _____ Gives rise to the lens
5. _____ Future optic nerve
6. _____ Differentiates into nonpigmented portion of the ciliary epithelium

7. _____ Tunica vasculosa lentis
8. _____ Ganglion cells of retina
9. _____ Hyaloid artery
10. _____ Surface ectoderm
11. _____ Congenital glaucoma
12. _____ Neuroectoderm

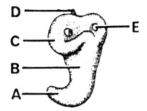

A. Conjunctival epithelium
B. Neuroectoderm
C. First pharyngeal pouch
D. First pharyngeal groove
E. Mesenchyme

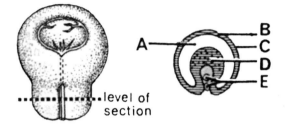

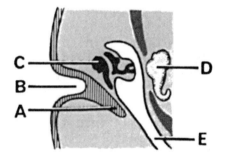

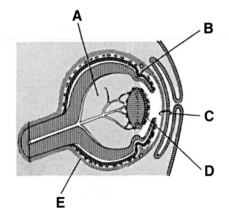

13. _____ Gives rise to a semicircular duct
14. _____ Absorption focus
15. _____ Endolymphatic duct
16. _____ Primordium of cochlea
17. _____ Saccular part of otic vesicle
18. _____ Gives rise to the spiral organ

19. _____ External acoustic meatus
20. _____ Sclera and choroid
21. _____ Has same origin as cornea
22. _____ Mastoid cells
23. _____ Bipolar cells of the retina
24. _____ Tympanic cavity

25. _____ Continuous with the pigmented epithelium of the retina
26. _____ Gradually obliterates
27. _____ Continuous with the neural layer of the retina
28. _____ Hyaloid vessels
29. _____ Continuous with the cranial meninges
30. _____ Contains axons of ganglion cells

31. _____ Derived from the first pharyngeal arch cartilage
32. _____ Gives rise to the utricle
33. _____ External acoustic meatus
34. _____ Meatal plug
35. _____ Derived from the tubotympanic recess
36. _____ Membranous labyrinth

37. _____ Only derived from surface ectoderm
38. _____ Ciliary body
39. _____ Develops from mesenchyme
40. _____ Composed of vitreous humor
41. _____ Cornea

## Answers and Explanations

1. **B** The external layer of the optic cup differentiates into the pigmented layer of the retina. The pigmented epithelium consists of a single layer of cells that reinforces the light-absorbing properties of the choroid membrane to reduce scattering of light within the eye.

2. **E**   The retinal fissure (optic fissure) develops on the inferior surface of the optic cup and along the optic stalk. The hyaloid blood vessels pass into the optic cup along this cleft and supply the lens and the developing neural layer of the retina.

3. **C**   The inner layer of the optic cup becomes the neural layer of the retina. It differentiates into the visual receptive portion of the adult retina. The inner layer of the optic cup also gives rise to the ciliary and the iridial parts of the retina.

4. **D**   The lens develops from the lens vesicle, a derivative of the surface ectoderm. The anterior wall of this vesicle becomes the anterior epithelium of the adult lens. Cells of the posterior wall lengthen to form lens fibers, which grow into and gradually obliterate the cavity of the lens vesicle.

5. **A**   The optic stalk, connecting the optic cup to the brain, becomes the optic nerve as axons of ganglion cells in the neural layer of the retina pass into the inner wall of the stalk. As a result of the continually increasing number of optic nerve fibers, the inner wall of the stalk increases in thickness and fuses with the outer wall, obliterating the lumen of the optic stalk.

6. **C**   Most of the inner layer of the optic cup becomes the neural layer of the retina. The anterior part becomes the nonpigmented portion of the ciliary epithelium (ciliary part of the retina) and the iridial portion of the retina. Toward the root of the iris, on the anterior surface of the ciliary processes, the cells of the inner layer of the cup gradually accumulate pigment granules.

7. **E**   The anterior part of the tunica vasculosa lentis, a vascular layer around the embryonic lens, is called the pupillary membrane. When the distal part of the hyaloid artery degenerates, the tunica vasculosa lentis, including the pupillary membrane, also degenerate. Remnants of this membrane often appear as tissue strands in normal eyes of infants, but these strands usually cause little disturbance of vision and tend to disappear in old age.

8. **B**   As the neural layer of the retina develops from the inner layer of the optic cup, the axons of ganglion cells in the retina pass into the inner wall of the optic stalk and gradually convert it into the optic nerve.

9. **D**   The hyaloid artery passes along the retinal fissure to the optic cup, where it supplies blood to the developing neural layer of the retina and to the embryonic lens. The distal portion of this artery usually degenerates, but the proximal part persists as the central artery of the retina. Persistence of the distal part of the hyaloid artery is a fairly common abnormality. It may persist in whole or in part, but it usually is not patent. The hyaloid arterial remnant appears as a thin line or thick cord in the vitreous humor.

10. **C**   The corneal epithelium is derived from the surface ectoderm. The lens functions as an inductor and influences the surface ectoderm to develop into the epithelium of the cornea. The substantia propria of the cornea is derived from mesenchyme.

11. **A**   Absence or incomplete development of the scleral venous sinus results in congenital glaucoma or buphthalmos. This abnormality usually is caused by recessive mutant genes, but sometimes it results from a maternal rubella infection during early pregnancy. The embryological basis of blockage or incomplete development of the scleral venous sinus is abnormal persistence of mesenchymal tissue in the angle of the anterior chamber. As a result of inadequate drainage of the aqueous humor through the canal, intraocular tension rises, the eye gradually enlarges, and the cornea becomes hazy. Retinal damage causes visual impairment.

12. **B**   The optic vesicle is an outgrowth of the brain. Hence, the retina and the optic nerve are derived from neuroectoderm of the embryonic brain. The adult structure of the retina and optic nerve shows a marked resemblance to the brain, and the coats of the eyeball and the optic nerve show resemblances to the coverings of the brain. The central artery and vein of the retina pass in the meningeal sheaths and are included in the anterior part of the optic

nerve. This relation is of clinical significance because an increase in pressure of cerebrospinal fluid around the optic nerve interferes with venous return from the eye, and edema of the optic disc (papilledema) results. This is an important indicator of an increase in intracranial pressure.

13. **C**   This flat, disclike diverticulum of the utricular portion of the otic vesicle is the primordium of one of the three semicircular ducts. They are attached to the utricle and later are enclosed in the semicircular canals of the bony labyrinth. The sensory areas (cristae ampullares), which develop in these ducts, respond to changes in the direction of movement of the head.

14. **E**   The central parts of the walls of the disclike diverticula from the utricular portion of the otocyst fuse and later disappear. Degeneration of tissue proceeds peripherally from the absorption focus, but peripheral portions of the diverticula remain as the semicircular ducts.

15. **D**   The endolymphatic duct appears as a hollow diverticulum from the dorsal utricular part of the otocyst. Its distal end expands to form the endolymphatic sac.

16. **A**   The cochlear duct develops as a tubular diverticulum from the saccular part of the otocyst. The cochlear duct grows and makes two and a half turns around the developing modiolus, a bony pillar or core that contains nerves and vessels. The coiled cochlear duct is called the membranous cochlea. It is contained in the bony cochlea, which develops from the surrounding mesenchyme.

17. **B**   The saccular part of the otic vesicle — the saccule — is an endolymph-containing dilation of the membranous labyrinth. The saccule contains a specialized area of sensory epithelium, the macula sacculi, and together with the macula utriculi signals the orientation of the head in space.

18. **A**   The spiral organ (of Corti) differentiates from cells in the wall of the cochlear duct. Ganglion cells of the eighth cranial nerve migrate along the coils of the cochlea and form the cochlear ganglion. Nerve processes grow from this ganglion to the spiral organ.

19. **D**   The external acoustic meatus is the adult derivative of the dorsal part of the first pharyngeal groove. It grows inward as a funnel-shaped tube until it reaches the endodermal tubotympanic recess, primordium of the tympanic cavity, tympanic antrum, pharyngotympanic (auditory) tube, and mastoid cells.

20. **E**   The sclera and choroid develop from mesenchyme that surrounds the optic cup. The mesenchyme differentiates into an inner vascular layer, the choroid, and an outer fibrous layer, the sclera. Toward the margin of the optic cup, the choroid becomes modified to form the cores of the ciliary processes, which consist chiefly of capillaries supported by delicate connective tissue.

21. **A**   The conjunctival epithelium, like the corneal epithelium, is derived from the surface ectoderm. The substantia propria of the conjunctiva and cornea consists of connective tissue derived from mesenchyme. The conjunctiva is a thin, transparent mucous membrane that covers the sclera and lines the eyelid. At the lid margin, the epithelium of the conjunctiva becomes continuous with the epidermis of the skin, another derivative of the surface ectoderm.

22. **C**   The mastoid cells begin to develop near term as the endodermal lining of the tympanic cavity, a derivative of the first pharyngeal pouch, induces erosion of the bone around the ear. The epithelium lining the mastoid cells formed by this process, called pneumatization, is derived from endoderm. Most mastoid cells develop after birth.

23. **B**   The bipolar cells of the neural part of the retina are derived from neuroectoderm of the brain. These cells are true neurons interposed between photoreceptor cells and ganglion cells.

24. **C**   The tympanic cavity develops from the expanded distal end of the tubotympanic recess, a derivative of the first pharyngeal pouch. The

tympanic cavity is a tiny epithelium-lined cavity in bone that communicates with the nasopharynx through the pharyngotympanic tube, another derivative of the first pharyngeal pouch.

25. **B**  The outer wall of the optic stalk is continuous with the outer wall of the optic cup, which gives rise to the pigmented epithelium of the retina.

26. **A**  The lumen of the optic stalk gradually obliterates as the optic nerve forms. As the number of axons of ganglion cells from the retina increases in the inner wall of the optic stalk, the lumen gradually disappears and the optic nerve forms.

27. **D**  The internal layer of the optic stalk is continuous with the inner layer of the optic cup, which gives rise to the neural layer of the retina. The internal layer of the optic stalk thickens as axons of ganglion cells pass through it on their way to the brain.

28. **E**  The hyaloid vessels supply blood to and return blood from the inner layer of the optic cup (future neural layer of retina) and the embryonic lens. The distal parts of these vessels usually degenerate and the remaining parts become the central artery and vein of the retina. When the retinal fissure closes, these vessels are incorporated into the optic nerve.

29. **C**  The sheath of the optic nerve is continuous with the meninges of the brain and with the choroid and sclera. When the optic vesicles develop as outgrowths of the brain, they carry the layers of the meninges with them.

30. **D**  The internal layer of the optic stalk contains axons of ganglion cells in the neural layer of the retina. About 1 million fibers eventually pass through the optic nerve, the adult derivative of the optic stalk. The optic nerve fibers are myelinated by oligodendrocytes instead of by Schwann cells because the optic nerve is comparable to a tract within the brain. The neuroepithelial cells in the walls of the optic stalk differentiate into oligodendrocytes and other neuroglial cells.

31. **C**  The malleus, one of the middle ear bones — auditory ossicles — is derived from the first pharyngeal arch cartilage. It develops by endochondral ossification of the dorsal end of the cartilage. The incus and stapes, the other two ossicles, are derived in a similar manner from the first and second pharyngeal arch cartilages, respectively.

32. **D**  The dorsal or utricular portion of the otic vesicle gives rise to the utricle. Like the saccule, it is a dilation of the membranous labyrinth that contains a specialized area of sensory epithelium, the macula utriculi. The utricle and saccule are sensors of head movements.

33. **B**  The external acoustic meatus is the adult derivative of the dorsal end of the first pharyngeal groove. This canal leads to the tympanic membrane, and its function (along with the auricle) is to collect sound waves, which cause resonant vibration of the tympanic membrane.

34. **A**  The ectodermal cells at the bottom of the developing external acoustic meatus proliferate and grow caudally as a solid epithelial plate — the meatal plug. Late in fetal life, the central cells of this plug degenerate, forming the inner part of the external acoustic meatus. Failure of the meatal plug to canalize results in atresia of the external acoustic meatus and deafness. This condition usually is caused by genetic factors.

35. **E**  The pharyngotympanic tube is derived from the tubotympanic recess, the derivative of the first pharyngeal pouch. This tube makes possible adjustments of pressure in the middle ear. When the tube opens during swallowing, the pressure in the middle ear is equalized with the atmospheric pressure.

36. **D**  The membranous labyrinth develops from the otic vesicle, a derivative of the surface ectoderm. It gives rise to the utricle, saccule, endolymphatic duct and sac, semicircular ducts, and cochlea. The internal ear, which has a dual function (hearing and equilibrium), consists of the membranous labyrinth derived from the otic vesicle. It is enclosed in the bony labyrinth derived from the surrounding mesenchyme.

37. **D**   The lens develops from the lens vesicle, a derivative of the surface ectoderm. The anterior wall of the hollow lens vesicle, composed of cuboidal epithelium, becomes the anterior lens epithelium. The tall columnar cells of the posterior wall of the vesicle lengthen to form highly transparent primary lens fibers that gradually fill the cavity of the vesicle. The corneal epithelium is derived from surface ectoderm, but its stroma is derived from mesenchyme, probably of neural crest origin.

38. **B**   The pigmented region of the epithelium of the ciliary body is derived from the outer region of the optic cup. It is continuous with the retinal pigment epithelium. The nonpigmented part of the ciliary epithelium represents the interior prolongation of the neural retina in which no neural elements differentiate. The ciliary muscle and connective tissue in the ciliary body develop from mesenchyme or early fibroblasts found at the edge of the optic cup.

39. **E**   The mesenchyme surrounding the optic cup differentiates into an inner vascular layer, the choroid, and an outer fibrous tunic, the sclera. The sclera develops from a condensation of the mesenchyme external to the choroid. It is continuous with the substantia propria of the cornea and with the dura mater that surrounds the optic nerve.

40. **A**   The vitreous body forms within the cavity of the optic cup, between the lens and retina. It is composed of vitreous humor, an avascular mass of intercellular substance. The primary vitreous forms from mesenchymal cells and hyaloid blood vessels. The mesenchymal cells are probably of neural crest origin. The primary vitreous becomes surrounded by a gelatinous secondary vitreous that probably arises from the inner layer of the optic cup. The secondary vitreous is formed from primitive hyalocytes, compact collagenous fibrillar material, and hyaluronic acid.

41. **C**   The lens induces formation of the cornea, which develops following separation of the lens vesicle from the surface ectoderm. The anterior surface of the cornea, which is covered by a stratified squamous, nonkeratinizing epithelium, forms from the surface ectoderm. The other layers of the cornea are probably derived from neural crest cells.

# Integumentary System

## Objectives

Be able to:

- Construct and label diagrams showing the development of skin, hair, nails, and sebaceous, sweat, and mammary glands.
- Write explanatory notes on each of the following congenital anomalies: ichthyosis, ectodermal dysplasia, athelia, amastia, polymastia, and polythelia.
- Discuss the development of teeth using labeled sketches to show the various stages of development.
- Define dental lamina, dental papilla, dental sac, epithelial root sheath, odontoblastic layer, odontoblastic processes, ameloblasts, and cementoblasts.
- Describe eruption of the deciduous and permanent teeth.
- Discuss the various causes of disturbances in enamel formation that result in enamel hypoplasia.

## Five-Choice Completion Questions

**Directions:** Each of the following statements or questions is followed by five suggested responses or completions. **Select the one best answer** in each case.

1. Which of the following structures is derived from mesenchyme?
   - A. dental papilla
   - B. fingernails
   - C. epidermis
   - D. sweat glands
   - E. tooth buds

2. Which structure is derived from surface ectoderm?
   - A. dental sac
   - B. dermal root sheath
   - C. arrector muscle of hair
   - D. odontoblastic layer
   - E. epithelial root sheath

3. Which cells are derived from the neural crest?
   - A. ameloblasts
   - B. odontoblasts
   - C. cementoblasts
   - D. melanoblasts
   - E. myoblasts

4. Most sebaceous glands develop as
   - A. downgrowths of the stratum germinativum
   - B. thickened areas of the epidermis
   - C. buds from the sides of hair follicles
   - D. downgrowths from the surface ectoderm
   - E. ingrowths along the glandular ridges

5. The ameloblasts of the developing tooth produce
   A. predentin
   B. dentin
   C. cement
   D. periodontium
   E. enamel

6. The odontoblasts of the developing tooth produce
   A. predentin
   B. dentin
   C. cement
   D. periodontium
   E. enamel

7. Which of the following congenital anomalies is common?
   A. hypertrichosis
   B. anonychia
   C. ectodermal dysplasia
   D. polymastia
   E. anodontia

8. Most congenital anomalies of teeth are caused by
   A. tetracyclines
   B. genetic factors
   C. rubella virus
   D. irradiation
   E. syphilis

9. "Birth marks" of flat, red cutaneous lesions were present on the face of a 3-month-old infant. These anomalies, diagnosed as angiomas of the skin, are caused by which of the following?
   A. increased melanocyte activity
   B. developmental defects of the dermis
   C. abnormal differentiation of the epidermis
   D. vascular anomalies
   E. excessive keratinization

10. Hypertrichosis was observed in the sacral region of a patient. This condition is associated with which of the following?
    A. spinal dermal sinus
    B. Arnold-Chiari defect
    C. absence of the sacral vertebrae
    D. spina bifida cystica
    E. spina bifida occulta

11. The teeth of an 8-year-old child were badly discolored, giving them a brownish yellow appearance, and the enamel was hypoplastic. This condition usually is associated with which of the following?
    A. congenital syphilis
    B. tetracyclines
    C. periodontal disease
    D. hypothyroidism
    E. dental papilla

12. An infant was diagnosed as having a disorder known as congenital ectodermal dysplasia. Which of the following would be present in the child?
    A. sparse body hair and no sweat glands
    B. thickened and highly keratinzed skin
    C. abundant sweat glands
    D. excessive hairiness
    E. natal teeth

13. In generalized albinism, which of the following usually shows some pigmentation?
    A. retina
    B. iris
    C. hair
    D. skin
    E. none of the above

14. Which of the following is *not* a hereditary disorder?
    - A. localized albinism
    - B. dentinogenesis imperfecta
    - C. hemangiomas
    - D. lamellar ichthyosis
    - E. polymastia

15. Which of the following is (are) involved in the growth of the lactiferous ducts after birth?
    - A. estrogens
    - B. progestogens
    - C. prolactin
    - D. growth hormone
    - E. all of the above

16. Albinism is a disorder of pigmentation due to a lack of melanin production by melanocytes. Regarding melanocytes and melanin, which of the following statements is correct?
    - A. Melanocytes are derived from mesenchyme.
    - B. Melanocytes produce melanin before birth.
    - C. Exposure to ultraviolet light decreases melanin production.
    - D. Cells containing melanin are present only in dermis.
    - E. Melanocytes produce melanin in the absence of the enzyme tyrosinase.

17. An infant was diagnosed with generalized albinism. The degree of pigmentation is regulated by
    - A. melanosomal p-protein
    - B. Wnt signaling
    - C. Sonic hedgehog (Shh) expression
    - D. retinoic acid
    - E. neural crest cells

18. Laboratory studies show that tooth bud formation is regulated by
    - A. Pax-6
    - B. Sonic hedgehog (Shh)
    - C. zinc-finger protein (ZFP)
    - D. Hox genes
    - E. fibroblast growth factor (FGF)

---

## Answers and Explanations

1. **A**  The dental papilla is a mass of condensed mesenchyme that invaginates the deep surface of the tooth bud. The dental papilla gives rise to the dentin and dental pulp.

2. **E**  The epithelial root sheath of the hair follicle and of the developing tooth is derived from the surface ectoderm. The dermal sheath (connective tissue) of the hair follicle, like the dental sac, is derived from mesenchyme.

3. **D**  Melanoblasts are derived from the neural crest, a derivative of the neuroectoderm. When the neural folds fuse to form the neural plate, some cells are not incorporated into it. These cells form a neural crest, which gives rise to the cells in the cranial, spinal, and autonomic ganglia; Schwann cells; melanoblasts; and cells of the suprarenal medulla.

4. **C**  All sebaceous glands develop as buds from the sides of the developing epithelial root sheaths of hair follicles, except those in the glans penis, eyelids, nostrils, anal region, and labia minora. In these sites, sebaceous glands develop as buds from the epidermis.

5. **E**  The ameloblasts differentiate from the cells in the inner enamel epithelium of the enamel organ. They produce enamel in the form of prisms (rods) and deposit it over the dentin. Each melanoblast produces one enamel rod, the structural unit of enamel. The ameloblasts degenerate after they have formed all the enamel and the tooth erupts. Thus, enamel is incapable of repair if it is injured by decay or injury.

6. **A**  The odontoblasts produce predentin and deposit it adjacent to the inner enamel

epithelium. Later, the predentin calcifies and becomes dentin. Hence, **A** is a better answer than **B**.

7. **D** An extra breast — polymastia — is quite common. About 1% of women have an extra breast or nipple. These usually develop just inferior to the normal breast, but they may appear anywhere along the line of the embryonic mammary ridges that run from the axillae to the inguinal regions.

8. **B** Most congenital anomalies of the teeth are hereditary (i.e., they are caused by genetic factors). The importance of genetic factors in tooth development and dental abnormalities is clearly demonstrated by studying the dentition in monozygotic twins. Tetracycline, an antibiotic, crosses the placenta and causes minor tooth defects (enamel hypoplasia) and discoloration of the deciduous teeth. Rubella virus, *Treponema pallidum* (the syphilis organism), and irradiation may also give rise to abnormalities to the teeth. Nutritional deficiency, diseases such as measles, and *high levels* of fluoride may damage the ameloblasts and cause defective enamel formation (enamel hypoplasia). Rickets resulting from a deficiency of vitamin D is, however, the most common cause of enamel hypoplasia. Abnormally shaped teeth are relatively common. Occasionally aberrant groups of ameloblasts give rise to spherical masses of enamel, called enamel pearls (drops), which often project from the side of the tooth.

9. **D** Angiomas of the skin or hemangiomas are localized vascular anomalies. A true hemangioma is a benign tumor of proliferating endothelium. These lesions include capillary angioma or cavernous hemangioma, the most common tumors found in infants and children.

10. **E** Hypertrichosis, or excessive hairiness, in the sacral area often is found in association with spina bifida occulta. It most commonly is seen over congenital melanocytic nevi. Hypertrichosis results from the development of supernumerary hair follicles and from the persistence of hairs that normally disappear during the perinatal period.

11. **B** Tetracyclines affect enamel formation and become incorporated into the developing enamel. These antibiotics should not be used during pregnancy and in children under age 12 because they interfere with metabolic processes that involve the ameloblasts.

12. **A** This is a rare hereditary disorder resulting from disturbances in the development of the epidermis and its appendages. The skin is defective and appears lax; often, other derivatives of the ectoderm, such as nails, hair, and sebaceous glands, may be partially or completely absent. Different clinical manifestations of ectodermal dysplasias have been recognized. Most likely, several modes of inheritance are possible for this condition.

13. **B** In cases of generalized albinism, the iris usually shows some pigmentation; however, the skin, hair, and retina lack pigment. Because of the lack of the enzyme tyrosinase, melanin is not produced by the melanocytes. In localized albinism, there is a lack of melanin in patches of skin, such as on the face, and/or of the hair.

14. **C** Hemangiomas are vascular anomalies, usually located on the face or neck. They are not an inheritable condition. Localized albinism and dentinogenesis imperfecta are autosomal dominant traits; lamellar ichthyosis is an autosomal recessive disorder; and polymastia is an inheritable condition.

15. **E** The main lactiferous ducts are formed at birth. Further growth and development of the lactiferous ducts in females occur particularly at puberty because of increased levels of circulating estrogens. Progestogens, prolactin, growth hormone, and corticoids also play a role. Increase in size of the female mammary glands during pregnancy is largely due to the rapid enlargement of the lactiferous ducts and deposition of fat.

16. **B** Only a few melanin-containing cells are normally present in the dermis. In the white race, the cell bodies of the melanocytes are usually confined to the basal layers of the epidermis. Melanocytes differentiate from

melanoblasts, which are derived from neural crest cells. Melanocytes appear in the developing skin between 40 and 50 days' gestation and begin to produce melanin before birth. Exposure to ultraviolet light results in an increased production of melanin. The enzyme tyrosinase is required for melanin synthesis.

17. **A** Neural cells give rise to melanoblasts. Wnt signaling regulates the differentiation of melanoblasts into melanocytes. MSH cell sur-

face receptor and melanosomal p-protein are genes that regulate the degree of pigmentation in melanocytes by controlling tyrosinase level and activity. Shh and retinoic acid are not involved in determining the degree of pigmentation.

18. **D** Laboratory studies indicate that Hox genes, Msx-1 and Msx-2 (transcription factors), play an essential role in the formation of the tooth bud, as well as in determining the shape and position of the tooth.

# Five-Choice Association Questions

**Directions:** Each group of questions below consists of a numbered list of descriptive words or phrases accompanied by a diagram with certain parts indicated by letters or by a list of lettered headings. For each numbered word or phrase, **select the lettered part or heading** that matches it correctly and then insert the letter in the space to the right of the appropriate number. Sometimes more than one numbered word or phrase may be correctly matched to the same lettered part or heading.

A. Dental pulp
B. Predentin
C. Dental sac
D. Enamel
E. Cement

1. _____ Periodontal ligament
2. _____ Odontoblasts
3. _____ Inner enamel epithelium
4. _____ Contains vessels and nerves
5. _____ Ameloblasts
6. _____ Inner cells of dental sac

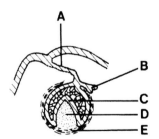

7. _____ Inner enamel epithelium
8. _____ Dental sac
9. _____ Dental lamina
10. _____ Dental papilla
11. _____ Bud of permanent tooth
12. _____ Part of enamel organ

A. Tetracyclines
B. Ameloblastic layer
C. Hair follicles
D. Neural crest cells
E. Epithelial root sheath of the
   developing tooth

13. _____ Melanocytes
14. _____ Induction of odontoblastic layer
15. _____ Lanugo
16. _____ Discoloration of teeth
17. _____ Sebaceous glands
18. _____ Fused layers of enamel epithelia
19. _____ Derived from inner enamel epithelium
20. _____ Derived from neural plate

## Answers and Explanations

1. **C**  The periodontal ligament is derived from the dental sac, a capsule-like structure that develops from the mesenchyme surrounding the tooth.

2. **B**  The odontoblasts derived from mesenchymal cells in the dental papilla (future pulp) give rise to predentin and deposit it adjacent to the inner enamel epithelium. Later, the predentin calcifies and becomes dentin.

3. **D**  Cells of the inner enamel epithelium adjacent to the dentin differentiate into ameloblasts. These cells produce enamel in the form of prisms (rods) and deposit it over the dentin.

4. **A**  The dental pulp derived from the mesenchymal dental papilla of the embryo contains the vessels and nerves of the tooth.

5. **D**  The ameloblasts are enamel formers. They produce long enamel prisms and deposit them over the dentin. Enamel formation begins at about 20 weeks in the deciduous teeth and continues in the permanent teeth until about age 16. If vitamin D is deficient during this period, the erupted surfaces of the teeth may be rough instead of smooth and shiny. The ameloblastic layer also induces the odontoblastic layer to form. Hence, if the ameloblasts do not differentiate normally (e.g., as in vitamin A deficiency), dentin formation is also affected.

6. **E**  The inner cells of the dental sac differentiate into cementoblasts, which produce cement (*L. cementum*) and deposit it over the dentin of the root.

7. **C**  The inner enamel epithelium of the enamel organ induces the adjacent mesenchymal cells in the dental papilla to differentiate into an odontoblastic layer. The inner enamel epithelium differentiates into ameloblasts, the enamel-forming cells.

8. **E**  The dental sac develops from the mesenchyme that surrounds the developing tooth. This capsule-like structure gives rise to cementoblasts, which form cementum, and to the periodontal ligament, which embeds in the cementum and the surrounding bony socket of the tooth. Thus, the periodontal ligament holds the tooth in its socket.

9. **A**  The dental lamina develops from the oral ectoderm and gives rise to the deciduous and permanent tooth buds.

10. **D**  The dental papilla, a condensation of mesenchyme, invaginates the tooth bud, giving it the appearance of a cap. The dental papilla gives rise to the dental pulp and to the odontoblasts, which form the dentin. There is some evidence that the mesenchymal cells that differentiate into odontoblasts are derived from the neural crest.

11. **B**  The tooth buds for the permanent teeth develop from continuations of the dental laminae. They begin to appear at about 10 weeks and lie lingual to the deciduous tooth buds.

12. **C**  The inner enamel epithelium is part of the enamel organ. Other parts are the outer enamel epithelium and the enamel reticulum. For a while, the enamel organ is attached to the oral epithelium by the dental lamina.

13. **D**  Melanocytes differentiate from melanoblasts, which are derived from neural crest cells. Melanoblasts migrate into the dermis during the early fetal period and soon enter the epidermis where they slowly differentiate into melanocytes. These cells produce melanin and distribute it to the epidermal cells after birth. Melanoblasts also migrate into the hair bulbs and differentiate into melanocytes. Melanin is distributed to the hair-forming cells before birth.

14. **B**  The ameloblastic layer induces the mesenchymal cells in the dental papilla adjacent to the inner enamel epithelium to differentiate into odontoblasts. If there is a deficiency of vitamin A, the ameloblasts do not differentiate properly. Consequently, there is abnormal formation of odontoblasts.

15. **C**  Lanugo is the soft downy hairs that are first produced by the hair follicles. These hairs are

chiefly shed before or right after birth and are replaced by coarser hairs that arise from new hair follicles.

16. **A** Tetracycline antibiotics are known to cause brownish yellow discoloration and fetal enamel hypoplasia if given to pregnant females or to children. If given after the eighth year, the third molar teeth are the only ones that may be affected because they are still developing.

17. **C** Most sebaceous glands arise as buds from the sides of the epithelial root sheaths of hair follicles, late in the second trimester of pregnancy. A few sebaceous glands develop from the epidermis, independently of hair follicles (e.g., in the eyelids and labia minora).

18. **E** The inner and outer enamel epithelia of the enamel organ come together and fuse in the neck region of the tooth, where they form the epithelial root sheath. This sheath grows into the mesenchyme and initiates root formation.

19. **B** The ameloblastic layer is derived from the inner enamel epithelium of the enamel organ. The ameloblasts produce enamel and deposit it over the dentin. As the enamel increases, the ameloblasts regress toward the outer enamel epithelium. Enamel and dentin formation begins at the tip (cusp) of the tooth and progresses toward the future root.

20. **D** Neural crest cells are derived from the neuroepithelium of the neural plate. When the neural folds fuse, some neuroectodermal cells at the lateral edges of the neural plate are not incorporated into the neural tube; these cells form the neural crest that gives rise to neural crest cells.

# Review Examination

## Introductory note:

The following multiple-choice questions are based on all chapters in this study guide and review manual. You should be able to answer these questions in one and a half hours. The key to the correct responses is on page 167.

## Five-Choice Completion Questions

**Directions:** Each of the following statements or questions is followed by five suggested responses or completions. **Select the one best answer** in each case.

1. Microscopic examination of a 14-day blastocyst revealed
   A. a primitive streak
   B. primary chorionic villi and lacunar networks
   C. a notochord
   D. a blastocyst surrounded by zona pellucida
   E. an intraembryonic coelom

2. Morphologically abnormal sperms are believed to cause
   A. monosomy
   B. congenital defects
   C. trisomy of the autosomes
   D. Klinefelter syndrome
   E. none of the above

3. The notochordal process lengthens by addition of cells from the
   A. notochord
   B. primitive streak
   C. notochordal plate
   D. primitive node
   E. primitive groove

4. During the early part of the fourth week, the rate of growth at the periphery of the embryonic disc fails to keep pace with rate of growth of the
   A. yolk sac
   B. neural tube
   C. embryonic coelom
   D. amniotic cavity
   E. primordial gut

5. Derivatives of the first pharyngeal pouch include
   A. tympanic antrum
   B. tubotympanic recess
   C. tympanic cavity
   D. pharyngotympanic tube
   E. all of the above

6. From the list of known human teratogens, the most likely cause of microcephaly is
   A. rubella (German measles)
   B. herpes simplex virus
   C. thalidomide
   D. therapeutic radiation
   E. *Toxoplasma gondii*

7. Which of the following would be inappropriate advice to give a woman who has just missed her menstrual period and may be pregnant?
   A. Obtain a vaccination against rubella infection.
   B. Avoid exposure to radiation whether for diagnostic or therapeutic purposes.
   C. Do not take any drugs that are not prescribed by a medical doctor.
   D. Stay away from people with infectious diseases.
   E. Eat a good-quality diet, and do not smoke.

8. An examination of the placenta and fetal membranes of male twins revealed two amnions, two chorions, and fused placentas. Twinning probably resulted from
   A. dispermy
   B. fertilization of two ova
   C. superfecundation
   D. fertilization of one ovum
   E. treatment with gonadotropins

9. Structures derived from the fourth pair of pharyngeal pouches include
   A. thymic corpuscles
   B. thymus gland
   C. superior parathyroid glands
   D. inferior parathyroid glands
   E. all of the above

10. The right auricle of the heart is derived from the
    A. primordial pulmonary vein
    B. sinus venosus
    C. right pulmonary vein
    D. sinus venarum
    E. primordial atrium

11. Which of the following structures is part of the second pharyngeal arch?
    A. facial nerve
    B. mandibular prominence
    C. Meckel cartilage
    D. primordium of malleus
    E. maxillary prominence

12. In humans, cleft lip, with or without cleft palate, usually results from
    A. riboflavin deficiency
    B. infectious diseases
    C. irradiation
    D. cortisone
    E. mutant genes

13. Which of the following is most likely to cause severe congenital anomalies in human embryos?
    A. cortisone
    B. potassium iodide
    C. aminopterin
    D. lysergic acid
    E. norethynodrel

14. The most distinctive characteristic of a primary chorionic villus is its
    A. outer syncytial layer
    B. cytotrophoblastic core
    C. villous appearance
    D. mesenchymal core
    E. cytotrophoblastic shell

15. A neonate with ambiguous genitalia was found to have chromatin-negative nuclei. Gonads were palpable in the inguinal canals. The phallus was short and curved (chordee). There was no family history of intersexuality. The most likely diagnosis is
    A. perineal hypospadias
    B. gonadal dysgenesis
    C. male pseudohermaphroditism
    D. female pseudohermaphroditism
    E. true hermaphroditism

16. Amniocentesis and amniotic fluid examination are most commonly used to
    A. diagnose chromosomal sex
    B. detect placental insufficiency
    C. determine the composition of the fluid
    D. detect chromosomal abnormalities
    E. diagnose a multiple gestation

17. Narrowing of the lumen in pyloric stenosis usually results from
    A. hypertrophy of the longitudinal muscular layer
    B. a diaphragm-like narrowing of the pyloric lumen
    C. persistence of the solid stage of pyloric development
    D. hypertrophy of the circular muscular layer
    E. fetal vascular accident

18. Which of the following cells produce pulmonary surfactant?
    A. type I alveolar epithelial cells
    B. type II alveolar epithelial cells
    C. alveolar macrophages (phagocytes)
    D. pulmonary epithelial cells
    E. endothelial cells

19. A neonate exhibits ambiguous external genitalia. Buccal smears show chromatin-positive nuclei. An elevated 17-ketosteroid output was detected. The most likely diagnosis is?
    A. gonadal dysgenesis resulting from chromosomal abnormalities
    B. female pseudohermaphroditism caused by maternal androgens
    C. congenital virilizing adrenocortical hyperplasia
    D. male infant with perineal hypospadias
    E. familial male pseudohermaphroditism

20. Anorectal agenesis usually is associated with a rectourethral fistula. The embryologic basis of the fistula is
    A. abnormal partitioning of the cloaca
    B. agenesis of the urorectal septum
    C. failure of fixation of the hindgut
    D. failure of the proctodeum to develop
    E. premature rupture of the anal membrane

21. Congenital heart disease most frequently results from
    A. maternal medications
    B. rubella virus
    C. mutant genes
    D. fetal distress
    E. genetic and environmental factors

22. The primordial germ cells are first observed in the
    A. dorsal mesentery
    B. primary sex cords
    C. gonadal ridges
    D. wall of the yolk sac
    E. mesoderm of the allantois

23. As the metanephric diverticulum grows it becomes capped by _____ mesoderm.
    A. splanchnic
    B. mesonephric
    C. metanephric
    D. somatic
    E. intermediate

24. The most common type of anorectal anomaly is
    A. anal stenosis
    B. anorectal agenesis
    C. ectopic anus
    D. anal agenesis
    E. persistent anal membrane

25. The most common cause of female pseudohermaphroditism is
    A. androgenic hormone ingestion
    B. adrenocortical hyperplasia
    C. maternal arrhenoblastoma
    D. testicular feminization
    E. maternal progestins

26. A fetus born prematurely during which of the following periods of lung development may survive?
    A. organogenetic
    B. canalicular
    C. pseudoglandular
    D. terminal sac
    E. embryonic

27. Exstrophy of the bladder often is associated with
    A. adrenocortical hyperplasia
    B. epispadias
    C. hypospadias
    D. urachal fistula
    E. chromosomal abnormalities

28. The most common congenital anomaly of the heart and great vessels associated with the congenital rubella syndrome is
    A. coarctation of the aorta
    B. tetralogy of Fallot
    C. patent ductus arteriosus
    D. atrial septal defect
    E. ventricular septal defect

29. The mesonephric duct in male embryos gives rise to the
    A. ductus deferens
    B. duct of Gartner
    C. ductules efferent
    D. duct of epoophoron
    E. rete testis

30. Hematopoiesis begins during the _____ week of development.
    A. third
    B. fourth
    C. fifth
    D. sixth
    E. seventh

31. The most common type of accessory rib is
    A. cervical
    B. sacral
    C. fused
    D. thoracic
    E. lumbar

32. Ameloblasts of the developing tooth produce
    A. predentin
    B. dentin
    C. cement
    D. enamel
    E. periodontium

33. Which of the following structures is derived from surface ectoderm?
    A. choroid
    B. membranous labyrinth
    C. extrinsic eye muscles
    D. sclera
    E. bony labyrinth

34. The myelin sheath of a peripheral nerve fiber is formed by
    A. mesenchymal cells
    B. neuroepithelial cells
    C. neurolemma (Schwann) cells
    D. neural crest cells
    E. microglia

35. A young mother gave birth to a child with ectrodactyly (lobster claw). The critical period of limb development for this defect after fertilization is from week
    A. 1 to 3
    B. 4 to 6
    C. 7 to 9
    D. 10 to 12
    E. 13 to 15

36. At birth, the inferior end of the spinal cord usually lies at the level of the _____ vertebra.
    A. first sacral
    B. third sacral
    C. first lumbar
    D. third lumbar
    E. twelfth thoracic

37. Structures derived from ectoderm include
    A. external acoustic meatus
    B. otic vesicle
    C. corneal epithelium
    D. lens
    E. all of the above

38. Cellular components of the retina derived from the internal layer of the optic cup include
    A. rod cells
    B. ganglion cells
    C. neuroglial cells
    D. bipolar cells
    E. all of the above

39. The myelin sheaths surrounding axons in the central nervous system are formed by
    A. neuroglial cells
    B. astrocytes
    C. oligodendrocytes
    D. microglial cells
    E. neurolemma cells

40. Myoblasts from the occipital myotomes give rise to muscles of the
    A. neck
    B. ear
    C. eye
    D. tongue
    E. pharynx

41. Most congenital anomalies of teeth are caused by
    A. rubella virus
    B. genetic factors
    C. tetracyclines
    D. irradiation
    E. syphilis

42. Conditions known to follow infection with cytomegalovirus or *Toxoplasma gondii* during the fetal period include
    A. mental retardation
    B. hydrocephaly
    C. microcephaly
    D. microphthalmia
    E. all of the above

# *Five-Choice Association Questions*

**Directions:** Each group of questions below consists of a numbered list of descriptive words or phrases accompanied by a diagram with certain parts indicated by letters or by a list of lettered headings. For each numbered word or phrase, **select the lettered part or heading** that matches it correctly and then insert the letter in the space to the right of the appropriate number. Sometimes more than one numbered word or phrase may be correctly matched to the same lettered part or heading.

A. Allantois
B. Primitive streak
C. Notochord
D. Blood island
E. Neural plate

43. _____ Gives rise to CNS
44. _____ Source of mesenchyme
45. _____ Rudimentary structure
46. _____ Develops in wall of yolk sac

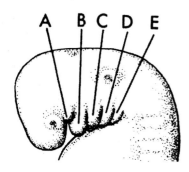

47. _____ Its muscle element gives rise to the muscles of facial expression
48. _____ Its cartilage forms a greater horn of the hyoid bone
49. _____ Its cartilage gives rise to a styloid process of the temporal bone
50. _____ Forms the inferior part of the face
51. _____ Gives rise to the lateral palatine process
52. _____ Supplied by the vagus nerve

A. Valve of the oval foramen
B. Partitions primordial atrium
C. Crista dividens
D. Oval foramen
E. Umbilical vein

53. _____ Its inferior edge directs blood to the left atrium
54. _____ Carries well-oxygenated blood to the fetus
55. _____ Remains of the septum primum
56. _____ Opening in septum secundum
57. _____ Early septum primum
58. _____ Part of septum secundum

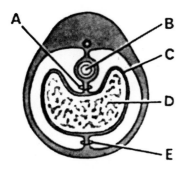

59. _____ Its free border contains the umbilical vein
60. _____ Embryonic site of hematopoiesis
61. _____ Derived from foregut and mid-gut
62. _____ Hepatoduodenal ligament

A. Scaphocephaly
B. Apical ectodermal ridge
C. Somites
D. Meromelia
E. Hemivertebra

63. _____ Exerts an inductive influence during limb development
64. _____ Craniosynostosis
65. _____ Partial absence of a limb
66. _____ Limb muscles
67. _____ Scoliosis
68. _____ Premature closure of sagittal suture

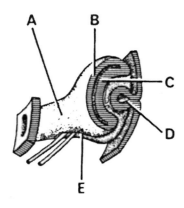

A. Neural crest
B. Alar plates
C. Basal plates
D. Neuroepithelium
E. Spinal ganglion cells

69. _____ Gives rise to the lens
70. _____ Future optic nerve
71. _____ Differentiates into nonpigmented part of the ciliary epithelium
72. _____ Becomes pigmented layer of the retina
73. _____ Retinal fissure
74. _____ Becomes specialized for sensitivity to light

75. _____ Gracile nuclei
76. _____ Form ventral gray columns
77. _____ Neuroglia
78. _____ Unipolar afferent neurons

# Key to Correct Responses

| | | | | | |
|---|---|---|---|---|---|
| 1. B | 14. B | 27. B | 40. D | 53. C | 66. C |
| 2. E | 15. A | 28. C | 41. B | 54. E | 67. E |
| 3. D | 16. D | 29. A | 42. E | 55. A | 68. A |
| 4. B | 17. D | 30. A | 43. E | 56. D | 69. D |
| 5. E | 18. B | 31. E | 44. B | 57. B | 70. A |
| 6. E | 19. C | 32. D | 45. A | 58. C | 71. C |
| 7. A | 20. A | 33. B | 46. D | 59. E | 72. B |
| 8. B | 21. E | 34. C | 47. C | 60. D | 73. E |
| 9. C | 22. D | 35. C | 48. D | 61. B | 74. C |
| 10. E | 23. C | 36. D | 49. C | 62. A | 75. B |
| 11. A | 24. B | 37. E | 50. B | 63. B | 76. C |
| 12. E | 25. B | 38. E | 51. A | 64. A | 77. D |
| 13. C | 26. D | 39. C | 52. E | 65. D | 78. E |

# Interpretation of Your Score

*Number of Correct Responses* | *Level of Performance*

| | |
|---|---|
| 70 – 78 | Excellent – Exceptional |
| 55 – 69 | Good – Superior |
| 43 – 54 | Average – Above Average |
| 37 – 42 | Poor – Marginal |
| 36 or less | Very Poor – Failure |

If you have not answered at least 50 of the questions correctly, determine the area where your knowledge is inadequate and read the chapters in your textbook related to these areas. When you feel confident that you understand this material, retry the examination until you can answer 70 of the questions correctly. *Do not try to memorize the answers* because this will not enable you to answer similar questions on USMLE or equivalent examinations.